CANNABIS & CBD

FOR HEALTH & WELLNESS

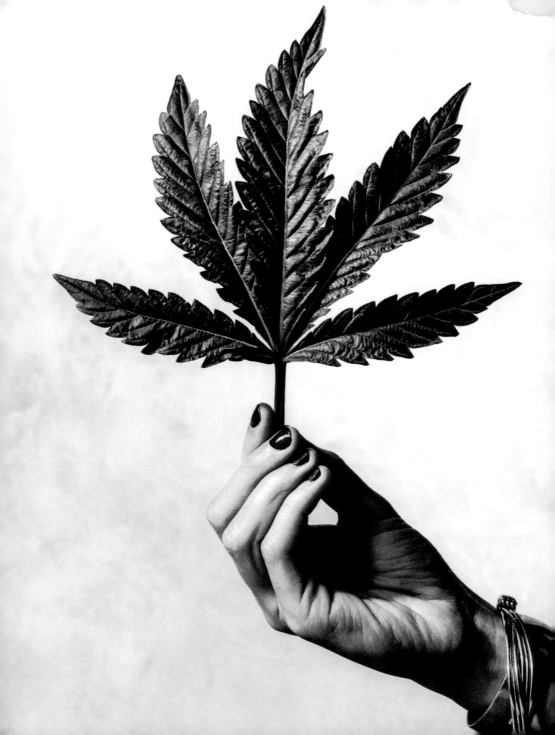

CANNABIS & CBD

FOR HEALTH & WELLNESS

An essential guide for using nature's medicine to relieve stress, anxiety, chronic pain, inflammation, and more

ALIZA SHERMAN
AND DR. JUNELLA CHIN

PHOTOGRAPHS BY ERIN SCOTT

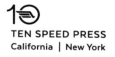

TEN SPEED PRESS
California | New York

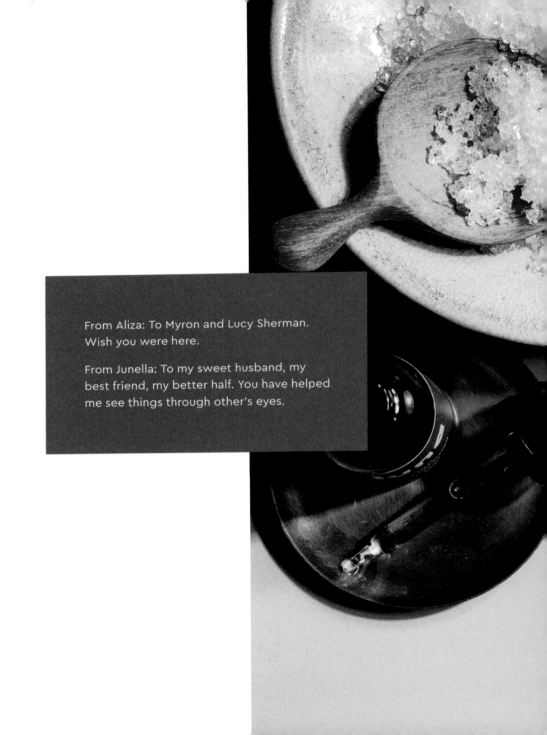

From Aliza: To Myron and Lucy Sherman.
Wish you were here.

From Junella: To my sweet husband, my
best friend, my better half. You have helped
me see things through other's eyes.

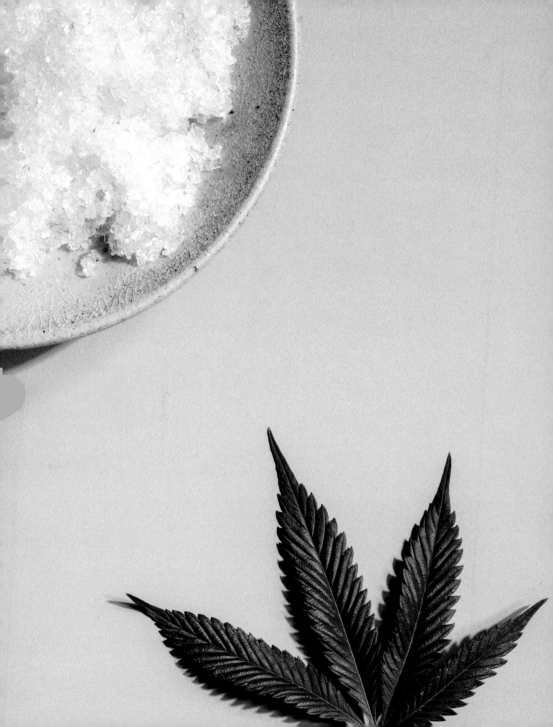

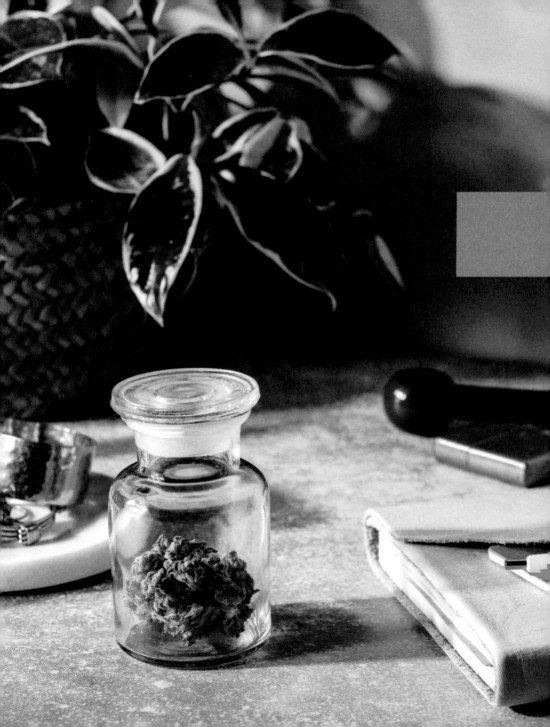

Contents

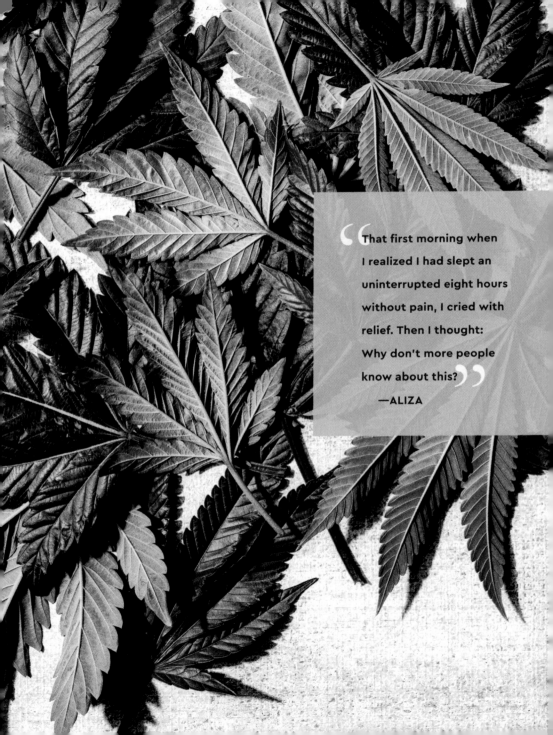

"That first morning when I realized I had slept an uninterrupted eight hours without pain, I cried with relief. Then I thought: Why don't more people know about this?"

—ALIZA

Introduction

We're here to tell you that cannabis is medicine. The anecdotal evidence gathered about the therapeutic benefits of cannabis is overwhelmingly positive. Research on cannabis—including cannabidiol, or CBD, which is contained within cannabis—is being conducted in many countries, with some research even taking place in the United States. The results are promising and support claims that cannabis can be used to reduce inflammation, relieve pain, and help people suffering from conditions ranging from epilepsy and Tourette's syndrome to Crohn's disease, multiple sclerosis, and rheumatoid arthritis.

And yet, in the United States, cannabis is still federally illegal, and many of us are nervous about looking into its health benefits. Did you look over your shoulder when you pulled this book from the shelf at your local bookstore or library? Or did you buy it online to avoid prying or disapproving eyes? If you did, you're not alone.

Many of us were taught to believe that cannabis is bad, unsavory, and dangerous. We might associate *pot* with stoners, *weed* with hippies, and *marijuana* with criminals. Luckily, attitudes about cannabis, and CBD in particular, are changing. According to the Pew Research Center, 62 percent of Americans say the use of cannabis should be legalized. You're probably seeing more human interest and news stories about cannabis and CBD in mainstream media about everything from cannabis-infused dinners to CBD beauty products. Depending on the legal status of cannabis and CBD in your city or state, you may be feeling more confident about exploring one or both for health and wellness. If you're living in a state that has not yet legalized cannabis, you can still do your homework and get ready for when your state does legalize or when you are visiting an adult-use (recreationally legal) state.

Cannabis can be used, with proper guidance from a medical professional, to replace pharmaceutical medications such as antianxiety drugs, SSRIs for depression, and opioids to address pain.

> "Cannabis changed the trajectory of my life. I would not have been able to finish medical school and become a doctor had it not been for cannabis treatment."
> —DR. JUNELLA CHIN

If you live in a state where physicians are not allowed to recommend cannabis, look online for naturopathic physicians or holistic nurses who may be open to recommending more alternative forms of medicine, or herbalists who are well versed in plant medicine. Also check the internet for services such as cannabis counseling and review the credentials of the counselors. Some nutritionists and other wellness professionals now offer cannabis consulting services. Always be very careful before substituting any prescribed medications with cannabis or CBD.

We both came to cannabis as women who were experiencing debilitating pain but were still plagued with fear and doubt about using it. We both changed our minds about cannabis over time because it helped us.

Our goal with this book is to help remove the remaining stigma associated with cannabis so that other people, like you, can gain health and wellness benefits from this ancient medicinal plant.

We'll provide tips and guidelines so you can begin using cannabis and CBD on your own, although we recommend that you see a medical care provider or a cannabis consultant for the most up-to-date information tailored to your specific needs. First, let us explain what brought us to cannabis.

JUNELLA'S STORY

At fifteen years old, I was diagnosed with ankylosing spondylitis (AS), a progressive type of arthritis that affects the spine, pelvis, hips, and back and causes extreme stiffness and nerve pain.

I spent my younger years trying conventional treatments—epidurals, narcotics, muscle relaxants, acupuncture, physical therapy—but the pain was unrelenting. By the time I got to medical school in San Francisco, I was having difficulty standing for long periods in the operating room. One of the attending physicians saw this and asked me about it. I told him I had AS but that I couldn't take the meds I needed for relief while doing rounds or while attending a four-hour hip-replacement surgery because they made me drowsy and foggy.

Here I was in a hospital surrounded by great medical minds, but I was disheartened to find nothing could help my condition. The attending physician pulled me aside and handed me a bottle containing a tincture. "This is marijuana," he told me, "but it won't make you high."

He didn't call it CBD oil. He just said it was a different type of cannabis plant. I was mortified but desperate. As a medical student, training to be a doctor, my first thought was, "You are offering me *pot*? You want to make me a drug addict?" The little brown dropper bottle smelled like a combination of alcohol, wet dog, and grass, and I didn't know what to think. To my amazement, the tincture worked very well. The pain and inflammation of my arthritis decreased dramatically, my ankylosing spondylitis stopped progressing, and my musculoskeletal health improved.

Even though California legalized medical marijuana in 1996, I didn't dare tell anyone I was using it. I was a young physician and didn't want to jeopardize my career. But once I got my health back, I decided to learn more about cannabis and how it helps manage pain and improve people's overall health and wellness.

Having suffered in pain for so long, I know what it feels like to say to your doctor, "I've tried everything and nothing has helped."

ALIZA'S STORY

When I first heard about cannabis being used for nonaddictive pain relief and insomnia relief in 2016, my first thought was, "If it is so effective, then why is it federally illegal?" I, like many people, bought into the idea that cannabis was dangerous and was made illegal to protect us all. Even though around seven states had already legalized cannabis by the time I began researching it for its therapeutic benefits, I was afraid to try it. At the same time, I was hopeful it could work for me.

After enduring two frozen shoulders and a few years of physical therapy in my late forties, by my early fifties I was in near-constant neck pain that my doctors attributed to years of computer use. The pain was keeping me up at night and limiting my mobility. I knew I needed to do something to address it when I couldn't turn my head while driving to look while changing lanes.

I also felt like a ticking time bomb, ready to explode from sleep deprivation and frazzled nerves. Despite my health issues, it took a while for me to regard cannabis as alternative medicine that could work alongside the homeopathy, chiropractic care, and acupuncture that I frequently turned to for pain management.

When I finally mustered the courage to try cannabis one night, the first thing I did was ground some indica flower (a variety of cannabis that produces relaxing effects) I purchased at a legal cannabis shop and tried vaping it (inhaling vapor versus smoke) with a vape pen. I immediately felt the acute pain in my neck subside after consuming only a small amount. For the first time in over a year, I slept through the night and woke up clearheaded and rested.

Once I experienced cannabis as effective medicine that worked without negative side effects, I knew I had to learn more about it and hopefully help others in the process. I am still cautious about using cannabis and even talking about it, but the more I hear from people that cannabis is helping them and changing their lives for the better, the more I know I'm doing the right thing.

IN THIS BOOK

Our goal is to guide you through your cannabis wellness journey or to help you guide a loved one with confidence. We learned over time, through our personal experiences and by doing our homework, that our fears about cannabis were unfounded. In chapter 1, we give a brief history of cannabis, outline why and how cannabis was vilified, and shed some light on how possessing and using a versatile medicinal plant became a crime.

You don't have to be a scientist or doctor to understand the science behind why cannabis is effective medicine. In chapters 2 through 5, we break down the elements of the cannabis plant and how they interact with our bodies, often drawing on scientific

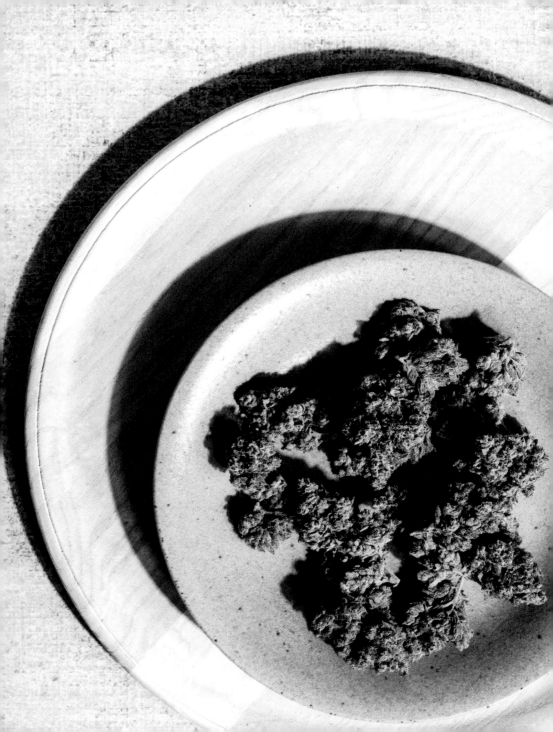

studies from countries such as Canada, Spain, the Netherlands, and Israel, where cannabis research is legal.

In chapters 6 and 7, we explain the different forms of cannabis, from the natural plant to extractions and infusions. We also delve into the different ways you can use cannabis: inhaling, ingesting, and applying. We explain dosages in chapter 8, in particular the use of small amounts, or *microdoses*.

Chapters 9 through 12 outline specific conditions, chronic and acute, that can be treated effectively with cannabis. Then we bring it all home, literally, in chapter 13, where we explain how to add cannabis to your medicine chest to improve your family's health and wellness.

We envision a day, not too far in the future, when cannabis will be legal across the country and as readily available to us as the herbal remedies and over-the-counter medicines we use regularly. The adage "Knowledge is power" is so true when it comes to cannabis and CBD. Better information about cannabis and CBD helps dispel myths and remove stigmas.

This book is the start of a new perspective on health and wellness and a new appreciation for the healing aspects of cannabis and CBD. We're excited to share accurate and clear information about cannabis with you and hope you share this book with everyone you know. Anyone can benefit from optimized health, and the more naturally we get there, the better!

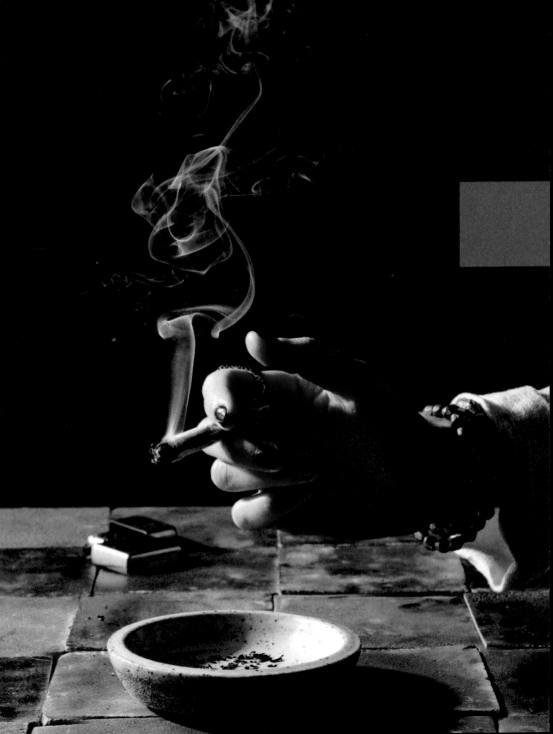

CHAPTER 1

A Brief History of Cannabis

The more we've learned about cannabis and why it was banned in the United States, the more we've come to realize that dishonesty—and greed—led us to the convoluted cannabis laws we have today. There are huge discrepancies between what our lawmakers tell us and what science and experience tell us about cannabis. A patchwork quilt of states has worked to individually overturn broken laws and return access to cannabis to people—particularly to people who need it for their health and well-being.

How did so many of us get to the place where we were—or are—afraid of cannabis and all that it represents? Why did we believe the misguided analogy of marijuana as a gateway drug? To understand this unfortunate evolution, let's go back in time, first to explore how cannabis was used throughout the centuries and then to examine the machinations that led the US government to ban cannabis.

CANNABIS AS AN ANCIENT HEALING PLANT

Cannabis was first used by ancient civilizations in spiritual and religious rituals and as a medicinal plant. The first cannabis plants are known to have come from Central Asia, particularly Mongolia and southern Siberia. Records from ancient civilizations show evidence of humans using cannabis in a number of ways, including:

1 Burning and inhaling the smoke
2 Crushing and mixing it with other herbs to form poultices, salves, or ointments
3 Cooking it and distilling it into tonics or beverages

Let's look at a timeline of the ancient and recent past of cannabis wellness. Please note that the following practices are not necessarily recommended today.

1800s BCE A plant thought to be cannabis was used for seizures and referenced in Sumerian and Akkadian tablets.

1700s BCE The Ramesseum Papyri, an Egyptian medical text, described using hemp to treat a patient's eyes.

1550 BCE An ancient Egyptian medical document called the Papyrus Ebers mentioned the use of cannabis to reduce inflammation. The document additionally noted grinding cannabis in honey and using it to "cool the uterus and eliminate its heat." Egyptian women also used cannabis as a medication to "cure wrath and grief."

1213 BCE Egyptian pharaoh Ramses the Great is believed to have used cannabis. In the 1980s, scientists found traces of cannabis in his mummified remains.

1000 BCE Ayurvedic and Arabic practices incorporated cannabis as an aphrodisiac and a pain reliever. The traditional Indian drink *bhang* is a mix of cannabis paste (made from the whole cannabis plant) and milk, ghee, and spices.

900 BCE Scythians, nomads of southern Siberia, used the smoke from burning hemp seeds for intoxication, according to Greek historian Herodotus.

100 CE A Chinese medical text, the *Shennong Bencaojing* or *Shennong's Materia Medica Classic*, mentioned the medicinal benefits of the flowers, seeds, and leaves of the cannabis plant.

200 CE In China, cannabis was used as an anesthetic during surgery. Surgeon Hua Tuo ground cannabis and combined it with wine for patients.

800 CE The *Al-Aqrabadhin Al-Saghir*, the first Arabic list of medicines with their effects and uses, described a cannabis-seed juice mixed with other herbs and taken intranasally to treat migraines and uterine pain, and to prevent miscarriage.

1600s Industrial hemp arrived in the American colonies and was grown at Jamestown, alongside tobacco, to produce rope, paper, and textiles. In 1639, the Massachusetts court passed a law requiring every household to plant hemp seed.

1700s Irish doctor William O'Shaughnessy wrote about the medical benefits of cannabis for rheumatism and nausea caused by cholera. American medical journals mentioned the use of hemp seeds and roots to treat health problems such as skin inflammation and incontinence. George Washington and Thomas Jefferson also grew hemp on their farms.

1800s Queen Victoria is said to have taken a monthly dose of cannabis prescribed by her physician to relieve menstrual cramps. In the United States, a medicinal syrup containing cannabis was used to provide relief from headaches, aid in better sleep, and stimulate appetite. It was also used during childbirth to start contractions and ease pain.

With all of the evidence over centuries of cannabis being used medicinally, how did it become illegal? The answer to that is due, in part, to the concerted efforts of a few powerful men who influenced how the public perceived cannabis, planting the seeds of stigma and driven by racial bigotry, political power grabbing, and greed.

WHY CANNABIS WAS MADE ILLEGAL

It wasn't until the early twentieth century that the view of cannabis shifted from versatile, natural medicine to dangerous drug. Change began to happen when Congress passed the Pure Food and Drug Act of 1906 leading to the formation of the US Food and Drug Administration (FDA). The law mandated that product labels list any of ten ingredients that were considered "addictive" and/or "dangerous." Cannabis was included on that list.

A Cannabis "Overdose" in Adults Isn't Deadly

Cannabis does not affect the parts of the brain that control breathing, heart rate, or body temperature. While receptors in our brains are affected by cannabis and create different reactions, including psychoactivity such as reducing anxiety or seizures or a psychotropic high, none of these receptors are in the brain stem and none of the reactions include deadly drops in breathing, heart rate, or body temperature as with alcohol or other controlled substances. In short, there are no recorded deaths directly attributed to a toxic level of cannabis in the body. According to David Schmader in his book *Weed: The User's Guide*, it would take consuming fifteen hundred pounds of cannabis (see page 15) in fifteen minutes to result in death. The schedule I listing of cannabis is puzzling. Even more confusing is how industrial hemp, a cannabis plant with 0.3 percent or less THC, is lumped in with cannabis plants grown for recreational or medical use. Moving cannabis down the list of controlled drugs and substances, or rescheduling (something some cannabis advocates are promoting), or regulating it like alcohol (as other advocates and lawmakers are recommending) may sound like good ideas, but regardless of how cannabis may be legalized or decriminalized, a lot of new challenges will come up before cannabis will become easily accessible to the masses.

After the Mexican Revolution of 1910, Mexican immigrants, who used the "marihuana" plant socially, brought it across the Mexican border into the United States. While some Americans, particularly high-profile and affluent individuals, used cannabis recreationally, others began associating cannabis with the minorities, including African Americans, who were using it. These associations were largely negative, and these attitudes were perpetuated by the media of the time.

During Prohibition, twenty-nine states outlawed cannabis along with alcohol. In 1933, Federal Bureau of Narcotics commissioner Harry Jacob Anslinger stated that cannabis did not make people violent, although he did say the desire for drugs caused some people to commit robberies to obtain money to purchase more. He would soon change his tune.

After Prohibition was lifted, Anslinger's position overseeing the Bureau of Prohibition was eliminated in 1937. He began a misguided campaign promoting the idea that cannabis caused some people to fly into a delirious rage, a drastic departure from his stance in 1933.

The federal government passed the Marihuana Tax Act in 1937 making the use of nonmedical cannabis illegal. The act was drafted by Anslinger and introduced by representative Robert L. Doughton of North Carolina. While this act did not criminalize the possession or use of marijuana, it did include penalties for violations of the outlined process of transferring the plant and paying taxes on it, resulting in a fine of up to $2000 and five years in prison.

Anslinger's attack on cannabis gave him a new battle to fight on behalf of the US government. Anslinger's cohorts who orchestrated campaigns to vilify cannabis included William Randolph Hearst, John D. Rockefeller, and Pierre du Pont—all men with investments in industries that could be threatened by the success of an industrial hemp industry that produced paper, biodiesel fuel, and a variety of other products.

The Controlled Substances Act (CSA) was passed in 1970, establishing the federal US drug policy to regulate the manufacture, importation, possession, use, and distribution of certain substances. Those substances were categorized by "schedules." President Richard Nixon repealed the Marihuana Tax Act in 1970, and cannabis was listed as a Schedule I drug. According to the US Drug Enforcement Agency (DEA), Schedule I substances are described in the following way:

▶ The drug or other substance has a high potential for abuse.

▶ The drug or other substance has no currently accepted medical use in treatment in the United States.

▶ There is a lack of accepted safety for use of the drug or other substance under medical supervision.

According to US federal law, no prescriptions may be written for Schedule I substances, and they are not easy to obtain for clinical use. Other substances listed in the Schedule I include psychoactive bath salts, MDMA, heroin, and LSD. For you the consumer, the best scenario is when cannabis is legal and there is some form of oversight to ensure quality and safety but it is readily available to you at an affordable price. Ideally, you'll also have better access to information about cannabis products, including ingredients, test results, and details on how to properly use them.

We're hopeful that the more people learn about the therapeutic benefits of cannabis, the more we will all advocate for legalization on terms that allow this natural medicine to become more widely used. One way to better understand how the cannabis plant works as medicine is to get to know the plant. In the next chapter, we'll look at the biology of cannabis.

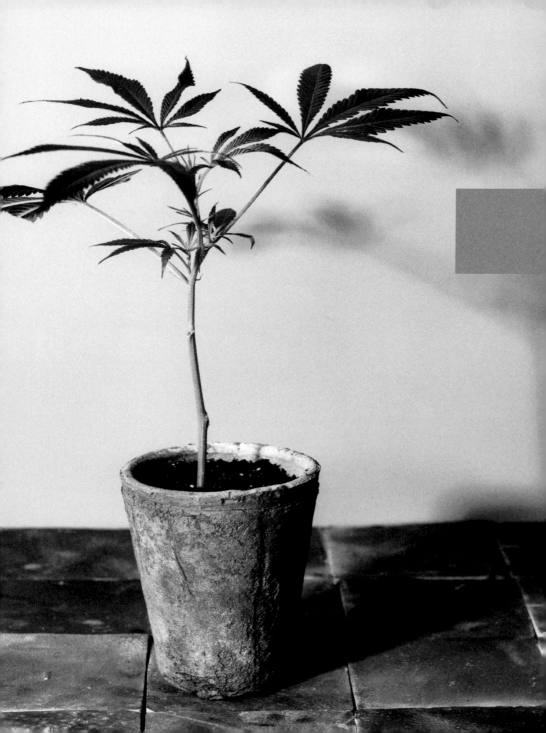

CHAPTER 2

The Cannabis Plant

To understand the therapeutic features of the cannabis plant, let's first get to know the plant in its natural forms.

CANNABIS, THE GENUS

If you remember middle school science, you probably learned about plant taxonomy. Plants, like all living creatures, are identified and named using a taxonomic naming system called binomial nomenclature for scientific classification. This systematic classification of plants is based on shared characteristics. Below is the basic taxonomy of the cannabis plant.

Kingdom: Plantae

Phylum: Angiosperma

Class: Dicotyledoas

Order: Rosales

Family: Cannabaceae

Genus: Cannabis

Species: *Cannabis sativa* L. marijuana

Subspecies: *Cannabis sativa* ssp. *indica*

Subspecies: *Cannabis sativa* ssp. *sativa*

Cannabis is the genus of flowering plant in the family Cannabaceae. Other genera in the Cannabaceae family are *Celtis*, more commonly known as hackberries or nettle trees, and *Humulus*, also known as hops. In this book, we will use the word *cannabis*, a more culturally accepted term than *marijuana*, *pot*, or *weed*, all of which have some negative connotations. Typically, when people refer to cannabis, they are speaking about the products derived from the plant itself rather than about the genus or species.

The two subspecies most commonly referenced and used are *Cannabis sativa* and *Cannabis indica,* and each contains numerous "strains," or genetic variants, including hybrids that blend both sativas and indicas. (There is a third subspecies— *Cannabis ruderalis*—based on unique traits, although it is less commonly used.)

Finding absolutely pure *Cannabis sativa* or *Cannabis indica* is not as likely as getting a hybrid or a blend that is mostly dominant in one subspecies but may have some genetic traces of another. The cannabis plant exhibits more diversity than other cultivated crops due to years of many different breeding and cultivation practices, particularly among black-market cannabis growers.

Different strains of cannabis are bred to contain different chemical makeups and potencies that, in turn, lead to different effects. Knowing more about the strain you're purchasing and consuming can help you anticipate the effects. Cannabis products derived from the indica subspecies are said to be more relaxing— providing a body high. Alternatively, a sativa strain might be more energizing—a head high. Note that some studies say strains don't matter as much when you ingest cannabis products because they change chemical form once they process through your liver. Identifying strains is useful when smoking or vaping cannabis.

Seek out specific strains—and pay attention to the *cannabinoids*, or chemical compounds, within them—to achieve more specific results. The most well-known compounds in the cannabis plant are THC (which produces an altered state of mind or high) and CBD (considered nonpsychotropic because it doesn't give you the high feeling). Note that CBD is often referred to as nonpsychoactive, but that isn't accurate. CBD and other cannabinoids in cannabis are *psychoactive* because they affect—and can protect—your brain, but not all of them are psychotropic so will not alter your mind's perceptions. (See chapter 4 for more details on *cannabinoids*.)

Cultivars or Chemovars: The Real "Strains"

While cannabis does grow wild in some places, the majority of the cannabis available to purchase has been cultivated to produce specific types of plants. These plant varieties produced during the cultivation process through selective breeding are called "cultivars"—short for "cultivated varieties." There are more than seven hundred cultivars of cannabis described to date.

Cannabis cultivars grown for medicinal or recreational purposes are commonly referred to as *strains*, although experts such as Dr. Robert Flannery, the first PhD in the United States with certified technical expertise in growing commercial cannabis, founder and CEO of Dr. Robb Farms, points out that the term *strain* is used to describe bacteria, not plants. While *cultivar* is the preferred term among growers and botanists, you'll most likely continue to encounter the term *strain* when researching and purchasing cannabis products. Popular strains of cannabis include Northern Lights, Gorilla Glue, Charlotte's Web, Sour Diesel, White Widow, and Kush. Scientists and doctors continue to discuss a different classification of cannabis to more clearly categorize the plant by *chemovars*. One way to do this is based on their *chemotype*, categorizing by the chemical compounds contained in each plant, and to breed plants for those specific makeups to try to get more consistency, such as by their terpene content. (See chapter 5 for information about terpenes.)

Some cannabis cultivars, such as the one commonly referred to as industrial hemp, are cultivated for their fiber or grown for seed that can be eaten raw or extracted for hemp oil.

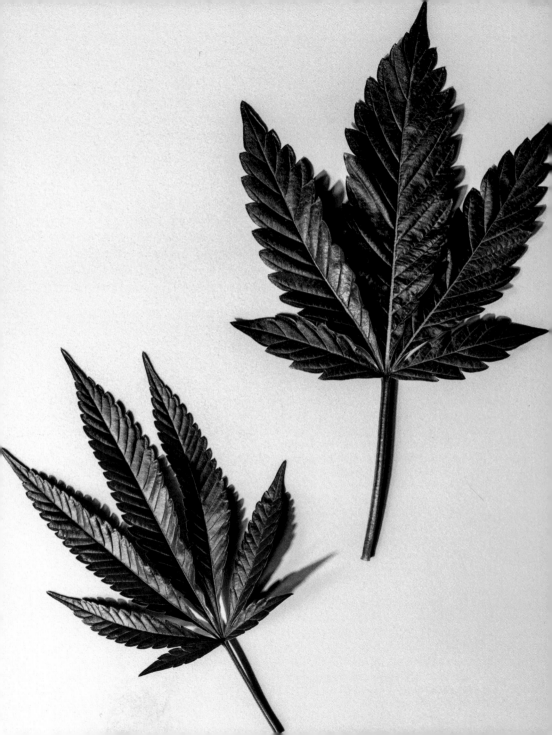

CANNABIS INDICA, THE SUBSPECIES

Cannabis indica is the shorter of the cannabis plant subspecies, growing to three to four feet tall with broad leaves and dense flower clusters. *Cannabis indica* plants have a shorter growing time than *Cannabis sativa*, eight to twelve weeks, which can explain why, in some cases, the supply of indica strains of cannabis at legal cannabis dispensaries or shops is more abundant than other strains.

Indica-dominant strains are more likely to produce what is referred to as a full-body high, characterized by deep relaxation and a feeling of sedation. A common description of the effects of *Cannabis indica* strains is "couch-lock," or being so relaxed you're stuck on the couch. Indicas can be effective to aid in sleep, reduce chronic pain, and relieve anxiety.

CANNABIS SATIVA, THE SUBSPECIES

Cannabis sativa is indigenous to eastern Asia but is now cultivated all over the world. Sativa is a taller plant than indica—growing up to twenty feet tall—with thinner, serrated leaves. Sativa plants take a longer time to become ready for harvesting, from between ten to sixteen weeks.

For most people, *Cannabis sativa* acts as a stimulant producing an energizing head high. People who are looking to remain alert and productive—or even creative—during the day may gravitate toward sativas, but they can keep some people up at night so are less likely to be used as a sleep aid.

CANNABIS RUDERALIS, THE SUBSPECIES

Cannabis ruderalis is a low-THC and low-resin subspecies of cannabis native to Central and Eastern Europe and Russia. Scientists dispute whether or not *Cannabis ruderalis* is its own unique subspecies or a subspecies of *Cannabis sativa*. Ruderalis is usually not grown for recreational use because of its low THC content but can be crossbred with other species of cannabis. In modern medicine, *Cannabis ruderalis* may be used to treat anxiety, epilepsy, and sclerosis and to increase appetite in cancer patients.

CANNABIS GROWN FOR CONSUMPTION

The cannabis we consume is obtained from the female (pistillate) cannabis plants. The male (staminate) plants are removed from the growing room during cultivation to allow the female plant to flower. If a female cannabis flower is pollinated, cannabinoid production stops, meaning the main chemical compounds within cannabis that make it unique and valuable for health and wellness are not present. When growing cannabis for consumption— either recreationally or medically—cannabis farmers work to cultivate female flowering plants to produce budding flowers at the flowering stage of the plants' growth cycle. Hemp plants are mostly male plants that do not flower.

When you are purchasing cannabis or cannabis-derived products, you may encounter a lot of descriptions of how the plant in question was grown; for example, full-sun, outdoor, or organic. As a consumer, look for "free of pesticides." If you're a fan of organically grown products, you may find some on the market to suit your preferences but usually at a higher price. Look for products that are free of heavy metals, particularly when purchasing hemp (see page 46).

The Role of Trichomes on Cannabis Plants

The leaves and buds of cannabis plants are covered with shiny, sticky hairlike features called *trichomes* that exist as a defense mechanism to protect the plant from insects, animals, fungus, ultraviolet rays, and wind. Trichomes are where cannabinoids and terpenes, the chemical compounds contained within the cannabis plant, are produced and accumulated. Trichomes house the compounds that contribute to the aroma of the plant matter, which can vary depending on the cultivar or chemovar. While the adjectives most often used to describe cannabis aroma are *skunky* or *musky*, compounds within trichomes can also release aromas reminiscent of citrus and pine, or flowers such as jasmine.

As cannabis plants begin to produce flowers, trichomes form along the outer surface of the plant. Cannabis farmers deliberately stress cannabis plants in a way that pushes trichome production without killing the plant. Once harvested, care is taken to maintain the trichomes on the plant matter as long as possible to preserve the full scope of compounds contained within them.

If you grind dried cannabis flower, a dustlike substance, known as *kief*, falls from the buds and is essentially dried trichomes. Some people like to capture kief and sprinkle it onto ground flower they are smoking or vaping to boost the plant matter's potency. Some cannabis grinders contain a compartment to capture and store kief.

Cannabis concentrates are produced using various extraction methods to pull the compound-rich trichomes from the plant material. Small amounts of concentrated cannabis extracts contain substantially more cannabinoids and terpenes than dried cannabis flowers and are more potent when consumed.

Cannabis goes through a number of stages from "seed to sale," and the stages depend on what final product is being produced. When you walk into a store, you are already far removed from the cannabis growing process, but you can ask any cannabis retailer, or *budtender*, questions about the growers and manufacturers they purchase from. A savvy retailer chooses cultivators and producers to work with, and receive product from, based on criteria other than price alone. These criteria often include organic growing processes, product purity, specific chemical compounds, and even the owner's and company's values. When you buy, ask questions and shop around until you find retailers who can give you satisfactory answers.

INDUSTRIAL HEMP

The hardy hemp plant can grow up to thirteen feet tall and tends to be easier to maintain than other cannabis plants because it is typically grown for seed production. Hemp leaves are thinner and more sparsely clustered than indica or sativa leaves. The main differences between cannabis and hemp are in their genetics and how they are cultivated (see "What Is the Difference Between Cannabis- and Hemp-Derived CBD?" on page 46 for more on this).

The hemp plant is part of the family Cannabaceae and genus *Cannabis* L. Hemp is *Cannabis sativa*, but this variety contains a lower percentage of THC. The cannabis plant grown for human consumption can contain up to 30 percent of the cannabinoid THC. Hemp has been selectively bred as an industrial plant to remove THC almost entirely—but not completely. To be legal in the United States, hemp plants and hemp-derived products must contain less than 0.3 percent of THC per dry weight. Hemp naturally contains more CBD than many cannabis plants bred for consumption. With legalization, cannabis cultivators are breeding new strains with higher CBD content to appeal to consumers who are becoming more aware of the compound's therapeutic benefits.

The plant we call industrial hemp has been used for centuries in a multitude of ways. The stalk of hemp plants are fibrous, and the fibers can be used to make rope, textiles, cosmetics, animal feed, and an array of other products, including bricks to build structures and fuel to run vehicles. Industrial hemp seeds are edible, and while they contain a negligible amount of CBD and absolutely no THC, they are rich in protein and omega fatty acids so have some nutritional value. You may already be eating hemp seeds in some granolas or nut and seed bars. You can buy hemp seeds in pouches at health food and grocery stores and sprinkle them on your cereal, yogurt, salads, or any dish where you might add sesame or chia seeds.

While many people consume cannabis recreationally for the high or relaxed euphoria, there is a growing number of people looking at cannabis as alternative medicine. In the next chapter, we'll discuss how chemicals within cannabis interact with chemicals in our bodies, resulting in therapeutic effects.

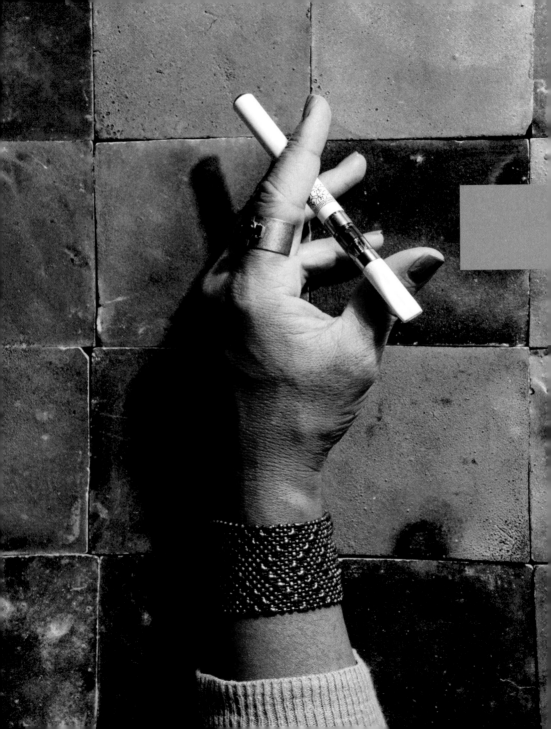

CHAPTER 3

Our Bodies, Our ECS

In this chapter, we'll introduce you to a system in your body that is an integral part of your health and well-being that you may not have ever heard of before now. To understand how cannabis works with your body and brain, think about some of the systems in our bodies that perform specific functions: digestive, circulatory, respiratory, and central and peripheral nervous systems, just to name a few. You most likely learned about these systems, to some extent, in science or health classes in school.

The human body contains another system that was discovered more recently, and has not been researched in the United States as extensively as it has been in other parts of the world. The system is called the endogenous cannabinoid system, more commonly referred to as the *endocannabinoid system*, or ECS for short.

WHAT IS THE ENDOCANNABINOID SYSTEM (ECS)?

Think of the endocannabinoid system, or ECS, as a system that lies over or interfaces with all of the other systems throughout your entire body. The ECS regulates both physical functions, such as movement, pain sensation, and immune responses, and cognitive or mental functions, like perception, mood, and memory.

While the name *endocannabinoid system* sounds like you have cannabis in your body, no cannabis is actually a part of this system. *Endogenous* means something produced naturally inside of the human body. The term *cannabinoid* alludes to cannabis only because these molecules were discovered in the 1990s during cannabis research.

Some scientists think that many human ailments and diseases—including pain, inflammation, multiple sclerosis, neurodegenerative disorders (Parkinson's disease, Huntington's disease, Tourette's syndrome, Alzheimer's disease), epilepsy, glaucoma, osteoporosis, and cancer—stem from an imbalance or weakness in the ECS and can be (or even have been) successfully treated by introducing phytocannabinoids (or plant cannabinoids) into the body.

Why might you not have heard of the ECS before this book? Scientific research on the ECS is relatively recent compared to the more extensive and long-standing research, often dating back to the 1800s, that we have on most other systems within our bodies. In the 1960s, scientists interested in centuries of evidence illustrating the medical uses of cannabis began to examine the plant more closely, trying to isolate and identify the various chemical compounds contained within it. A few decades later, scientists were interested in how the cells of mammals responded to chemicals within cannabis plants. In 1988 and 1992, two cannabis receptors were discovered and found to be keys to an entire system, the ECS. We cover more about those receptors in a bit.

The endocannabinoid system modulates different systems in your body, including the release of hormones related to stress and even reproductive functions such as fertility. Overall, a well-functioning ECS works to bring your internal systems into balance. The technical term for this type of balance within the human body is *homeostasis*. When you're sick, your body's internal endocannabinoid system jumps into gear to help put things back in order. Your ECS is key to establishing and maintaining your overall health and well-being.

Scientists who are studying the ECS consider this particular system to be most important because of how it resides within and affects every part of the body. Simply put, there isn't any physiological process that is not affected by the ECS. The ECS comes into play when we eat, sleep, relax, exercise, and have sex, as well as during pregnancy, while giving birth, and even when nursing a baby. Your ECS also helps regulate your immune system.

There are three parts that make up the endocannabinoid system:

1 Receptors that detect molecules outside of cells and activate signals inside of cells

2 Endogenous cannabinoids or endocannabinoids—the human body's internal cannabinoids

3 Enzymes, technically called degradative enzymes, that break down our endocannabinoids after they perform a particular function, like reducing anxiety, to stop the ECS from running amok

Endocannabinoids are present in cell membranes throughout the body. In a sense, endocannabinoids are your own body's internal cannabis molecules without the cannabis. Even if you never consume cannabis, you still have endocannabinoid molecules inside of you. If you do consume cannabis, phytocannabinoids in the cannabis plant will bind with receptors in your body and can stimulate, supplement, and nourish your ECS, promoting balance, improving health, and effectively managing conditions and treating diseases.

INTRODUCING OUR CELLULAR GATEKEEPERS

Before we continue talking about the ECS, we want to introduce you to receptors in your body called G-protein coupled receptors (GPCRs), which act as gatekeepers of molecular signals. Not to get too technical, but GPCRs take stimuli from outside of cells in your body and convert them to signals inside your cells. GPCRs are involved in every important physiological process within our bodies, from immune system function to regulating our metabolism to how we taste and smell food.

GPCRs are so important in the medical field that more than 40 percent of all pharmaceutical drugs target them. Common drugs that target GPCRs include triptans for migraines, beta blockers for hypertension, albuterol for asthma, cimetidine and ranitidine for stomach ulcers, loratadine for allergies, and fentanyl and oxycodone for pain. GPCRs are also targets for cancer drugs on the market and in development.

Why are we telling you about GPCRs? Because two critical parts of the ECS are GPCRs—called CB1 and CB2—and both respond positively to cannabis.

CB1 AND CB2 RECEPTORS: LOCKS UNLOCKED BY CANNABIS

Both CB1 and CB2 receptors are located throughout our bodies. In fact, CB1 is the most abundant GPCR in our central nervous system. How does this relate to cannabis? Because, like pharmaceuticals, cannabis targets CB1 and CB2, it stands to reason that cannabis can work as medicine. Cannabis has been shown to have fewer negative side effects than typical pharmaceuticals. Cannabis also has an extreme "lack of toxicity," meaning you cannot take a lethal dose of cannabis—it is physiologically impossible (see page 13).

So where are CB1 and CB2 receptors located?

▶ CB1 receptors are found mostly in the brain and central nervous system, connective tissues, glands, and organs. When cannabis is consumed, phytocannabinoids within the plant bind to the CB1 receptors in your brain, leading to psychoactivity (affecting the brain) such as reducing anxiety, as well as the psychotropic or mind-altering effect of feeling high.

▶ CB2 receptors are found mostly in your immune system and peripheral nervous system. When CB2 receptors are activated, they can address inflammatory conditions and help boost your immune system response.

Think of the CB1 and CB2 receptors as locks within your body. So what are the keys that unlock these receptors to enhance physiological functions? The keys are both naturally occurring endocannabinoids in our ECS as well as phytocannabinoids within the cannabis plant. Phytocannabinoids are not unique to cannabis. These chemical compounds also occur in plants such as echinacea, a common alternative medicine used as an immune booster and sold in health food stores across the country.

The most well-known phytocannabinoids—or cannabinoids—in cannabis are THC and CBD, and they interact with our ECS by binding to (THC), or affecting (CBD), our CB1 and CB2 receptors. The bottom line is our bodies respond positively to cannabis. We'll go into a lot more detail about endocannabinoids and phytocannabinoids in chapter 4.

By the way, research in 2016 found that other chemical compounds within plants interact with our ECS, including carrot, kava, ginger, and black pepper. While these plants don't seem to have cannabinoids per se, they affect how our bodies process cannabinoids. Pepper, for example, can quickly reduce the effects of THC, a helpful thing to remember if you ever consume too much cannabis and feel uncomfortably high—just chew on a peppercorn!

So far, scientists have identified at least 113 cannabinoids in the cannabis plant, more than any other plant in nature. Cannabis should be considered a superfood because of all the therapeutically beneficial chemical compounds it contains. With so many different cannabinoids in cannabis, there are seemingly infinite ways this plant can be used to enhance our health and wellness. We're only beginning to understand the science behind how and why cannabis works for us.

To sum things up, the ECS modulates functions throughout the body using receptors, namely CB1 and CB2, that are affected by cannabinoids and other compounds found in cannabis as well as other plants we consume. In the next chapter, we'll explore specific cannabinoids contained in the cannabis plant and explain their effects on us.

Discovering the ECS

An organic chemist in Israel, Raphael Mechoulam, isolated THC in 1964, but it wasn't until 1988 that scientist Allyn Howlett and American pharmacologist William Devane at St. Louis University Medical School in Missouri discovered the first cannabinoid receptor, type 1 or CB1, in a rat's brain. CB1 was found to mostly reside in the central nervous system. In 1992, Mechoulam, Devane, and Lumír Ondřej Hanuš isolated the first endocannabinoid from a pig's brain at Hebrew University in Jerusalem, Israel. They named this chemical compound anandamide, based on the Sanskrit word for "bliss," *ananda*. A study in 1993 led by Sean Munro at the University of Cambridge identified the second cannabinoid receptor, cannabinoid receptor type 2 or CB2. CB2 receptors are found mostly in the cells of our immune system. A third receptor, GPR55, was discovered in 1999, but research still needs to be done to uncover its functions. While the ability to research cannabis is greatly hindered in the United States by federal law, US studies of the ECS and the effects of cannabis on the human body continue. They are studied more extensively in other countries, including Israel, the United Kingdom, the Netherlands, Italy, and Canada.

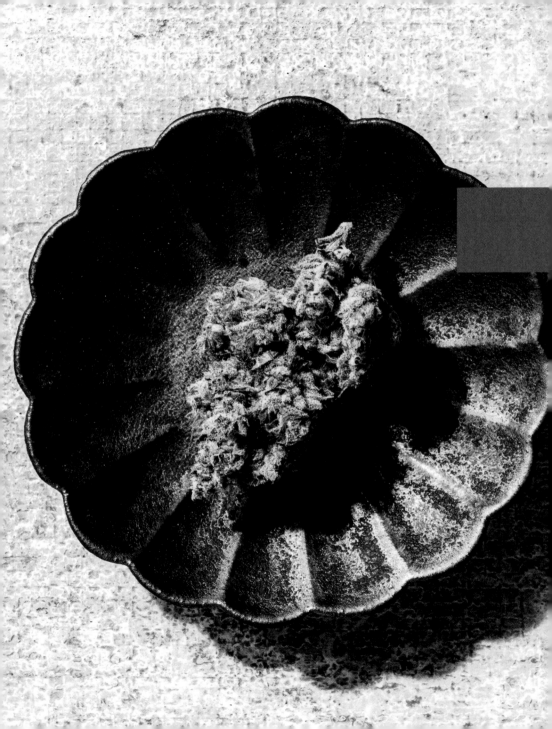

CHAPTER 4

Cannabinoids— Key Elements in Cannabis

The cannabis plant is densely packed with chemical compounds that set it apart from other plants. We've mentioned that cannabis boasts more than a hundred phytocannabinoids, or plant cannabinoids. For comparison, echinacea, black pepper, black truffles, and cacao each contain a few phytocannabinoids or phytocannabinoid-like chemicals or enzymes that affect the ECS similarly, but less effectively, than cannabis. For example, chocolate and black truffles naturally produce anandamide, the "bliss molecule," when you consume them.

What do plant cannabinoids do, and how do they interact with our bodies? As we mentioned in the previous chapter, these compounds bind to receptors called CB1 and CB2 in our endocannabinoid system. The various cannabinoids outlined in this chapter interact with each other and enhance the cannabis plant's therapeutic benefits. When you hear people talking about using "whole-plant" cannabis extracts, they are referring to the benefits of keeping the related compounds within cannabis together, as close to the way they are present in the natural plant, so they interact more as nature intended. The intricate composition of the whole plant is greater than the sum of its parts, like a musical symphony versus a solo instrument playing.

The research behind cannabinoids in cannabis is still in its infancy, but the results of the preclinical studies are promising and reveal potential therapeutic benefits such as those listed in this chapter. The diagram on the next page illustrates the most common cannabinoid compounds and their relationship to each other, starting with CBGA, the raw acid form of CBG.

CBGA is converted into the acid forms of THC, CBD, and CBC—which are THCA and CBDA (more on these forms on pages 38 to 44). Heat between 220°F and 245°F (104°C and 118°C) must be used to convert these acids to the cannabinoids on the next level in the diagram—THC, CBD, CBC, and other active cannabinoids. When someone smokes or vapes cannabis, they are heating or warming the plant matter or concentrated form to activate it or *decarboxylate* ("decarb") it. Appliances on the market such as Levo and Ardent's Nova help you easily make cannabis oils and butters at home by decarboxylating cannabis flower with less mess than the old method of cooking it in the oven or a slow cooker or on the stove.

Age and exposure to the elements can naturally convert the active cannabinoids into those on the bottom level of the diagram. Cannabinoids at the bottom levels can still contribute to the health and wellness benefits of cannabis. For example, CBN can be used as a sleep aid.

Without access to a lab for testing decarbed cannabis flower you produce at home, you really can't accurately predict or measure how much of any cannabinoid is present in what you have produced. Trying to produce CBN by exposing your cannabis flower to air and light, for example, degrades the product. You could end up producing an excess of CBN, and consuming too much CBN could result in an unwanted psychoactive effect: paranoia.

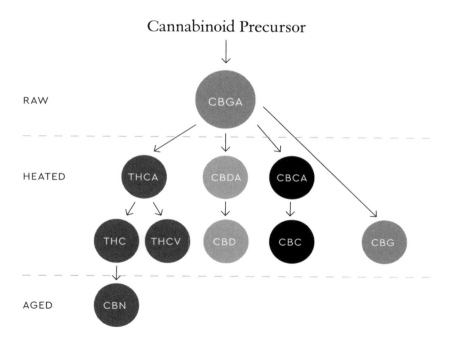

Cannabinoid Precursor

RAW — CBGA

HEATED — THCA · CBDA · CBCA

THC · THCV · CBD · CBC · CBG

AGED — CBN

When you go shopping for cannabis flower and cannabis-derived products, ask for testing results or visit the manufacturer's website to see if they break down the chemical makeup, including cannabinoid content. Not every manufacturer or retailer makes this information available, but a good budtender finds out product details for customers. Keep shopping around until you get the details you need to make purchasing decisions based on potential therapeutic benefits tied to specific cannabinoids.

Following are the most common cannabinoids found in the cannabis plant along with some of the health benefits outlined in a variety of scientific and medical studies, some of which are listed in the Selected Bibliography starting on page 161. Some cannabinoids are lesser known or studied at this time, but scientist believe they, too, will be revealed to have health-related benefits.

CBGA (CANNABIGEROL ACID)

CBGA is considered the "mother" cannabinoid because it is ultimately converted into all other cannabinoids (see the diagram on page 37). The cannabis plant naturally produces CBGA first as a raw chemical. When CBGA is exposed to heat, either from UV light or a heat source, an enzymatic process is triggered that converts CBGA into THCA, CBDA, or CBCA (the A signifies "acid"). Heat, in turn, converts those acid forms of cannabinoids into other cannabinoids, such as THC, CBD, and CBC. CBGA is not psychotropic.

Potential Therapeutic Benefits of CBGA: Treating glaucoma, fighting cancer, serving as an antibacterial agent, stimulating appetite, preventing bladder dysfunction, and reducing inflammation, including decreasing inflammatory bowel disease.

THCA (TETRAHYDROCANNABINOLIC ACID)

THCA, the acid form of THC, exists in the raw cannabis plant. To convert it into a form that can be absorbed into the human bloodstream and bind to our ECS receptors, it first needs to be decarboxylated. Because the live cannabis plant contains only THCA, you don't get high juicing raw cannabis leaves.

Potential Therapeutic Benefits of THCA: Reducing inflammation, protecting neurons in the brain, reducing nausea, and increasing appetite.

THC (TETRAHYDROCANNABINOL)

THC is one of the "Big Six" cannabinoids, a designation given to the six most well-known, researched, and medically utilized cannabinoids that also tend to be the most prominent in the cannabis we consume. THC is one of the few cannabinoids that produces psychotropic, or mind-altering, effects. THC binds to CB1 receptors in our brains, releasing dopamine and other chemicals that create altered moods, perceptions, and cognition. When you purchase dried cannabis flower or concentrates such as oils, heat converts the THCA to THC. Other cannabis products, such as edibles and tablets, contain decarboxylated THCA, or THC, so are already activated to provide effects.

Potential Therapeutic Benefits of THC: Reducing pain and inflammation, easing nausea and vomiting, increasing appetite, controlling diarrhea, protecting neurons in the brain, aiding sleep, and treating Post Traumatic Stress Disorder (PTSD).

THCV (TETRAHYDROCANNABIVARIN)

THCV, counted as one of the Big Six cannabinoids, is said to be more psychotropic than its root compound, THC, but for shorter durations of time. THCV has a higher boiling point than THC—428°F (220°C) versus 314.6°F (157°C)—so it requires higher heat to convert. THCV thwarts the common notion that cannabis gives you the munchies by actually suppressing your appetite.

Potential Therapeutic Benefits of THCV: Suppressing appetite; reducing pain, panic attacks, and insulin resistance; regulating blood sugar levels; stimulating bone growth; and reducing tremors, motor control issues, and brain lesions associated with Alzheimer's and Parkinson's diseases.

CBN (CANNABINOL)

CBN is another Big Six cannabinoid. When THC degrades due to exposure to air and light, CBN is formed. CBN is prominent in old, dried cannabis flower. Consumed in large quantities, CBN can produce paranoia, something you might experience after smoking low-quality, improperly stored pot. Storing cannabis in airtight containers makes it last longer and slows the process of naturally produced CBN. Darker or colored containers can also slow CBN production. When dried cannabis is crispy or completely brown, that could be a sign that it is older or was stored improperly, and may make you sleepy or paranoid or both.

Potential Therapeutic Benefits of CBN: Acting as a sedative, working as an antibiotic and antibacterial, reducing convulsions, and stimulating bone cell growth. It also shows promise as an analgesic.

CBD (CANNABIDIOL)

CBD is also one of the Big Six cannabinoids. Think of CBD as a complementary compound to THC but without the mind-altering aspects. CBD is psychoactive, meaning it affects your brain, but in protective and healing ways such as reducing seizures and treating post-traumatic stress disorder.In 2018, the World Health Organization (WHO) determined that there is no public health risk or abuse potential for CBD.

CBD nutritional supplements and beauty products are becoming popular in the marketplace and can be found in places such as drugstores, health food stores, neuropathic natural medicine clinics, and in some dispensaries, depending on local or state cannabis and CBD laws. CBD can be derived from cannabis plants grown for consumption; but to be legal in the United States, CBD must be extracted from industrial hemp plants and contain only trace amounts of THC—under 0.3 percent. CBD doesn't bind to our cannabinoid receptors on its own but can influence the binding action of other compounds in our ECS to CB2 receptors, supporting and boosting our immune system and reducing inflammation.

CBD can affect how THC binds with our CB1 receptors, reducing the psychotropic effects of THC while still allowing us to get the therapeutic effects of both. CBD can be infused in virtually any product, including skin care and hair care, beverages and foods, tinctures, and tablets. CBD is not psychotropic like THC, meaning it doesn't alter your mind's perceptions. CBD takes longer to build up in your system before you experience results so don't expect immediate effects when using CBD. How CBD affects you will vary based on potency and the form you consume.

Potential Therapeutic Benefits of CBD: Reducing pain, inflammation, nausea, seizures, and anxiety; and aiding sleep.

Whole Plant/Full Spectrum vs. Isolates: The Entourage Effect

As cannabis products evolve, licensed manufacturers manipulate the plant to extract, concentrate, or even isolate compounds including cannabinoids and terpenes. In some cases, compounds are removed and then certain ones are reintroduced in an attempt to produce different effects, such as isolating CBD for its anti-inflammatory properties. The terms used to describe an extraction process that involves the entire plant are *whole-plant* or *full-spectrum* extracts.

Because the cannabinoids in the cannabis plant work together, complementing, enhancing, or modulating each other, some experts think that keeping them together in their most natural form is more effective medicine, an interactive process called the *entourage effect*. An example of the entourage effect can be seen with the two major compounds of the cannabis plant, THC and CBD. When taken together, CBD modulates and neutralizes the psychotropic effects of THC. The combinations of the plant compounds are antagonistic, meaning they work against or opposite one another. At the same time, they are synergistic, meaning they also work well together, with their opposite behavior complementing each other. Even a small amount of THC can help the CBD molecules affect your CB1 receptors, increasing therapeutic benefits throughout your body.

The opposite of whole-plant extracts are *isolates*, where single cannabinoids are isolated. Note that there are also *distillates* that are formed through a chemical process that separates the cannabinoids and terpenes by heating basic cannabis oil to a boiling point. Each cannabinoid and terpene in cannabis has a distinct boiling point at which it is released. Distillates still have some cannabinoids or terpenes, depending how you distill the cannabis oil. Refining the oil further gets you to a crystalline isolate with no other compounds present.

Within the cannabis industry there is debate over whether or not isolating cannabinoids deprives consumers of the full therapeutic benefits of cannabinoids working together. Some companies that produce and sell full-spectrum CBD products promote the potential benefits of the entourage effect. Think of "whole plant" as similar to "whole foods." Eating a whole carrot is better for you than buying the beta-carotene supplement at the vitamin store because it is rich in more complex nutrients than a processed, isolated compound. Companies producing isolates—including pharmaceutical companies—point to the ability to zero in on and control specific effects as well as dose with more precision when using isolates. Further research will tell us more about which form is most beneficial, although it may depend on what effects you're trying to achieve.

CBC (CANNABICHROMENE)

CBGA converts to CBCA, which in turn, converts to CBC. CBC is one of the Big Six cannabinoids and the third most abundant next to THC and CBD. Nonpsychotropic, CBC has anti-inflammatory properties that become more effective when combined with THC, an example of the natural interactions between cannabinoids in cannabis where one enhances the other.

Potential Therapeutic Benefits of CBC: Fighting cancer, reducing pain and inflammation, promoting healthy brain function, stimulating bone tissue growth, acting as an antibiotic and antifungal, and inhibiting acne.

CBG (CANNABIGEROL)

CBG is also nonintoxicating. Its chemical parent is CBGA, from which all other cannabinoids are naturally produced. CBG typically occurs in much lower amounts than other cannabinoids in the cannabis plant. While it is considered a minor cannabinoid, it is still one of the Big Six. Research conducted in Europe showed CBG to be antibacterial and effective against resistant bacteria strains such as methicillin-resistant *Staphylococcus aureus* (MRSA).

Potential Therapeutic Benefits of CBG: Treating glaucoma, decreasing inflammation in inflammatory bowel syndrome, fighting cancer, protecting neurons in the brain, preventing bladder dysfunction, and fighting antibiotic-resistant bacteria.

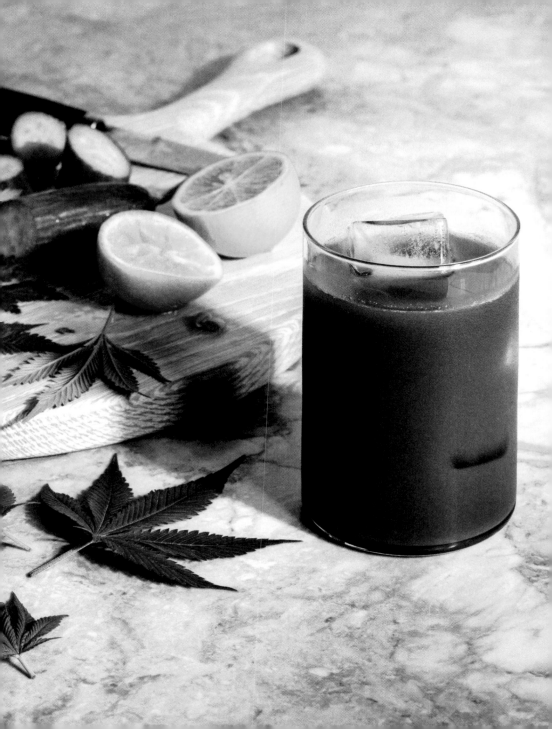

What Is the Difference Between Cannabis- and Hemp-Derived CBD?

Not all CBD is created equal, and not all CBD is sourced from the same version of the plant subspecies *Cannabis sativa*. The hemp plant is grown differently than the cannabis plant we consume. While they are both *Cannabis sativa*, hemp plants are low-resin plants, meaning they don't naturally produce the sticky substance that is usually present in woody plants. The hemp plant contains CBD but negligible amounts of THC, less than 0.3 percent.

THC is formed in resin glands located on the buds and flowers of the female cannabis plant. Because industrial hemp isn't cultivated to produce buds or flowers, it doesn't produce high THC content. Industrial hemp is grown to make paper, clothes, fiber, and food. Cannabis plants produced for consumption are female flowering plants containing higher amounts of naturally produced resin with higher THC content and a wider range of medicinal and intoxicating uses.

The 2019 Farm Bill made it legal to grow industrial hemp in the United States and legal to sell industrial hemp–derived CBD products grown in the US as well as abroad. However, it does not cover CBD derived from cannabis that is grown for consumption, even if the THC is removed. CBD derived from high-THC plants falls in a legal gray area, even in states where cannabis is legal.

Hemp plants are classified as phytoextractors, meaning they can remove dangerous compounds from soil such as heavy metals, or hyperaccumulators, meaning they can grow in soils containing dangerous compounds and absorb them into their tissues. Hemp was planted at the site of the Chernobyl nuclear meltdown to help decontaminate the soil at a rapid rate. Land developers often plant hemp around old, abandoned toxic factory sites for the phytoextraction. Think of the hemp plant as a natural environmental vacuum cleaner, sucking pollutants out of the soil.

Given this fact of nature, when purchasing hemp-derived CBD, be aware of the possibility that it could contain contaminants. Seek out products that are third-party-tested for solvents, heavy metals, pesticides, and fungus. Also, look at the extraction method used in the production of the hemp-derived CBD you buy and use. Extraction methods using propane, hexane, pentane, and butane are cheaper but can leave toxic residue. Ethanol extraction is considered a safer method for extracting CBD from plant matter as is "supercritical CO_2 extraction," which uses carbon dioxide under high pressure with cold temperatures. When shopping at a dispensary, ask the budtender, manager, or customer service rep about the extraction methods used in products you are considering. Look for the least toxic or solventless extraction method. If you can't get answers to your questions where you're purchasing, review manufacturer websites or contact the companies directly, especially if they don't publicly list their extraction process.

From an environmental standpoint, industrial hemp typically produces a small amount of hemp-derived CBD during the extraction process, so more plants are required than with CBD-rich cannabis. Legalizing cannabis for CBD extraction would be easier on the environment and produce less waste.

As we've explained in this chapter, cannabinoids are the chemical components of cannabis that are the keys to unlocking your CB1 and CB2 receptors, activating and modulating your endocannabinoid system to optimize your health and wellness. If you think cannabis is chock-full of cannabinoids, wait until you learn in the next chapter about the multitude of terpenes contained within the plant.

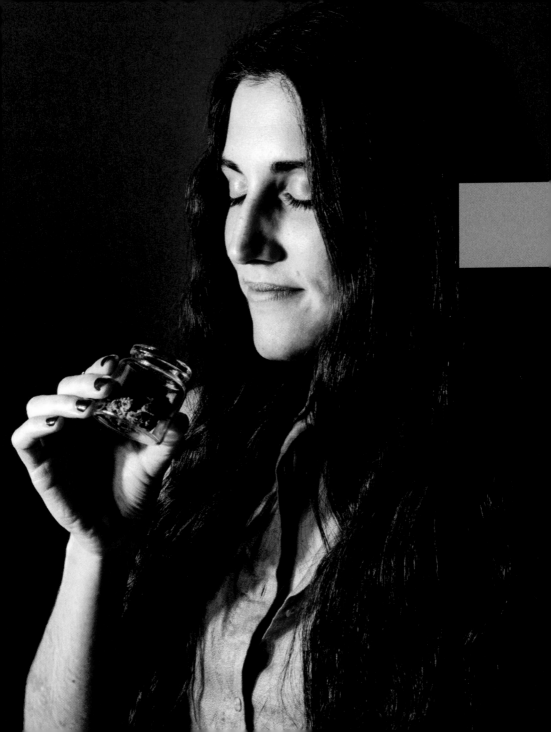

CHAPTER 5

Terpenes— The Aromatherapy of Cannabis

Cannabinoids are not the only compounds within cannabis that affect our ECS and interact with our bodies and brains, although they are the only ones that actually bind to our CB1 or CB2 receptors. *Terpenes* are hydrocarbons (made up of hydrogen and carbon molecules) and organic compounds that are present in medicinal plants, flowers, fruits, and vegetables. Cannabis contains a wide array of terpenes that can enhance or modify how cannabinoids act or interact, making them an important part of the overall mix of compounds that affect how cannabis works within us.

Terpenes within the essential oils of medicinal plants are part of a plant's natural way of repelling predators and attracting pollinators. Terpenes produce color, smell, and taste, so the red in a tomato, the citrus taste of an orange, and the woodsy astringent smell of pine needles are produced, in part, by terpenes. Look in your kitchen spice cabinet. Cinnamon, cloves, rosemary, ginger root, thyme, and basil, to name a few, all get their distinct aromas and flavors from terpenes. In general, terpenes are considered safe to consume and to use topically because they have low toxicity, and they are often used as food additives for color, taste, and smell. Some, such as the linalool in lavender, are even used in perfumes for their aroma or, as in the alpha-pinene found in rosemary, in natural skincare products for their antibacterial properties.

If you think about aromatherapy, the therapeutic use of aromatic plant extracts and essential oils, cannabis can be used in similar ways when it is rich in terpenes. While the cannabis plant contains more than two hundred different terpenes, most cannabis products on the market contain significant amounts of only a handful of terpenes. Each cannabis strain contains varying percentages of specific terpenes, and the therapeutic effects of the cannabis products you purchase and consume will vary based on the terpene makeup known as the "terpene profile."

In this chapter, we outline some benefits of the most common terpenes found in cannabis and CBD products, including topicals, foods and beverages, tinctures, tablets, and other manufactured forms. In the past, cannabis growers and manufacturers did not always pay attention to terpene content. Today, with savvier consumers, many are growing and producing for specific terpene profiles to address specific conditions such as pain or inflammation or to achieve specific effects such as focus, elation, relaxation, or high energy.

Terpenes are what give cannabis an earthy, musky, sometimes skunky odor that people might mistakenly attribute to THC. The terpene profile of cannabis, as with any plant, herb, spice, or food, contributes to how it smells and even how it tastes, including subtle hints of citrus, fruit, or flowers. To some, the smell of cannabis is unpleasant, while others find it appealing and are able to detect the more nuanced aromas of various terpenes. Terpene-rich cannabis has a pungent aroma while cheaper, lower-quality, or older pot tends to have less smell. Depending on how you consume cannabis, you may be able to detect the terpenes, particularly when you smoke or vape it and release the oils—or resin—within the plant matter.

When consumed, terpenes and cannabinoids within cannabis work together to produce specific effects in the human body and brain. This interaction is part of the entourage effect, described previously on page 42. Terpenes present in a particular strain of cannabis can greatly influence the medicinal qualities and reactions, enhancing or tempering the effects of the cannabinoids. When terpenes in cannabis are heated, they combine to form a chemical-reaction cascade that may also direct how your body responds to the cannabinoids.

Keep in mind that a strain or cultivar that is high in a terpene you're looking for—such as pinene for alertness—might also contain a terpene that will offset it, like the more sedating myrcene. In the same way you might use lavender essential oils in your bath to relax or drink peppermint tea to pep up, different plants with different terpenes produce specific effects when applied, inhaled, or ingested. Look at the overall terpene profile to seek out complementary terpenes. Another thing to remember is that cannabis flower comes from a plant, not a laboratory, so its chemical makeup can vary from crop to region to cultivation method.

To find these specific terpenes, just as with cannabinoids, you can ask a budtender for products with particular terpene profiles or review manufacturer websites where components or ingredients are listed. Some dispensaries provide test results for cannabis flower, breaking down terpene content, while others do not because it requires an additional testing fee to measure them. Smart manufacturers or retailers know that consumers like you are looking to tap into the health benefits of cannabis and are interested in the contents of the products they buy and consume.

Here is a breakdown of the potential features, both externally and internally, of terpenes found in cannabis and other plants. Comparing cannabis to more familiar plants shows how and why cannabis is able to provide therapeutic benefits such as aromatherapy. Note that the strains listed are known to contain specific terpenes, but double-check testing results to make sure. Cross-breeding can change the chemical makeup of each plant.

ALPHA-PINENE AND BETA-PINENE

Also found in rosemary, pine needles, dill, and basil.

AROMA: Pine trees, turpentine

TOPICAL USE: Antiseptic, analgesic, antibacterial, antifungal, anti-inflammatory

INTERNAL USE: Relieves symptoms of asthma (bronchodilator), anti-inflammatory

STRAINS: Jack Herer by Sensi Seeds, OG Kush

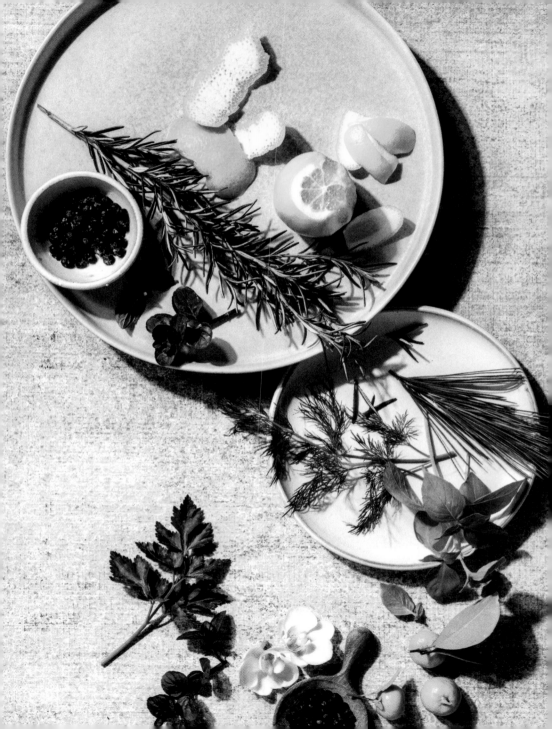

BETA-CARYOPHYLLENE

Also found in black pepper, cloves, hops, basil, rosemary, and oregano. Binds directly to the CB2 receptor (immune system) similarly to a cannabinoid.

AROMA: Peppery, spicy

TOPICAL USE: Anti-inflammatory, analgesic

INTERNAL USE: Antioxidant, reduces muscle spasms and pain from inflammation, potentially suppresses cancerous tumor growth

STRAINS: OG Shark, Trainwreck

GERANIOL

Also found in geraniums, lemon, and tobacco.

AROMA: Roselike, fruity

TOPICAL USE: Mosquito repellent, relieves neuropathy, antifungal

INTERNAL USE: Anti-inflammatory, anticancer, neuroprotectant, antiviral, antispasmodic, antioxidant

STRAINS: Amnesia Haze, White Shark, OG Kush

HUMULENE

Also found in cloves, basil, hops, sage, ginseng, and coriander.

AROMA: Earthy, woodsy

TOPICAL USE: Anti-inflammatory, antibacterial, analgesic, wound healing

INTERNAL USE: Pain relief, appetite suppressant

STRAINS: Master Kush, Skywalker OG

LIMONENE

Also found in juniper, peppermint, rosemary, and the rinds of citrus.

AROMA: Citrusy

TOPICAL USE: Antifungal, antibacterial, aids in absorption of terpenes transdermally and through mucous membranes

INTERNAL USE: Immune system support, antidepressant, antianxiety, antioxidant, anticancer, anti-inflammatory, can treat gastrointestinal issues and heartburn

STRAINS: Headband, Super Lemon Haze

LINALOOL

Also found in lavender.

AROMA: Floral, citrusy

TOPICAL USE: Antimicrobial, pain reduction

INTERNAL USE: Anticonvulsant, antidepressant, sedative, immune system support

STRAINS: LA Confidential, Skywalker OG

MYRCENE

Also found in hops, basil, mango, thyme, bay leaves, and lemongrass.

AROMA: Musky, clovelike, fruity

TOPICAL USE: Antiseptic, antibacterial, antifungal, enhances transdermal absorption

INTERNAL USE: Reduces inflammation, sedative, appetite aid, nausea relief

STRAINS: Warlock CBD, White Widow

OCIMENE

Also found in mint, parsley, pepper, basil, kumquats, mangoes, and orchids.

AROMA: Woodsy, herbal

TOPICAL USE: Antifungal, antiseptic, antibacterial

INTERNAL USE: Antifungal, antiviral, decongestant

STRAINS: Golden Goat, Strawberry Cough

TERPINEOL

Also found in lilac, pine trees, lime blossoms, and eucalyptus sap.

AROMA: Floral, piney, smoky

TOPICAL USE: Anti-inflammatory, antibiotic

INTERNAL USE: Sedative, antianxiety, antitumor, antioxidant, antibiotic, antimalarial

STRAINS: Fire OG, Skywalker OG

TERPINOLENE

Also found in nutmeg, conifers, apples, cumin, lilacs, and allspice.

AROMA: Piney, floral, herbal

TOPICAL USE: Antifungal, antibacterial

INTERNAL USE: Antioxidant, anticancer, sedative when inhaled, used to treat Crohn's disease and ulcerative colitis

STRAINS: Durban Poison, Jack Herer

VALANCENE

Also found in Valencia oranges.

AROMA: Citrusy, sweet

TOPICAL USE: Mosquito and tick repellent

INTERNAL USE: Anti-inflammatory

STRAINS: Tangie, Agent Orange

Due to the way cannabis used to be grown on the black market, not all cannabis plants are rich in terpenes. Cultivating cannabis for a richer terpene profile is a more recent endeavor as cannabis consumers become more discerning and many more people are seeking out therapeutic benefits from their cannabis.

When purchasing legal cannabis, ask to see the test results of the products you are considering, particularly the breakdown and percentages of terpenes. The average terpene content varies from strain to strain, but typically myrcene and alpha-pinene are the most abundant, followed by beta-caryophyllene, limonene, and a few others. Abundant for myrcene could mean up to 8 milligrams per gram, falling to about 2 milligrams per gram or less for the rest of the terpenes. Terpene content is only a fraction of the chemical makeup of any given strain, but when a particular terpene shows up in test results, consider its effects when determining what to purchase.

Depending on the form of cannabis you purchase and consume, the terpenes may have been removed in an extraction process or, in some cases, eliminated altogether or reintroduced to promote a particular effect. In manufactured products, look for the list of ingredients or mentions of terpenes, if there are any. Cannabis flower and edibles made from butters or oils infused using cannabis flower should contain more of the naturally occurring terpenes in the plant.

Remember we are talking about plant matter versus synthetically produced medications, so there may be a lot of variation in percentages of cannabinoids and terpenes in cannabis flower and concentrates. Manufactured cannabis products can get closer to precise and consistent chemical makeup. Not all legal cannabis shops showcase the terpene profiles of their products because terpene testing can be an extra expense, but knowing which terpenes are present—and prevalent—can help you find a cannabis strain that best suits your needs. A well-trained budtender can help you decipher test results and point you toward products that may be right for you.

Don't ask a budtender to diagnose you or prescribe a particular product. It is against the law for a budtender to provide medical advice. Instead, ask for specific cannabinoids or terpenes you want based on the lists we've compiled in this and the previous chapter. You can say, "I'm looking for a sleep aid" or "I'm trying to address neck pain" as a lead-in to "I'd like something rich in myrcene" or "I'd like something with analgesic cannabinoids and terpenes." The rest of the process of finding the ideal cannabis for your needs is up to you. Experiment with different strains and forms and keep a detailed journal (see page 100) until you get the effects that you desire.

As the cannabis market matures, companies are manipulating plants to produce products in different forms for more dosing precision or to zero in on certain effects. How a cannabis product is manufactured can lead to a more specific chemical makeup that can better serve your needs. In the next chapter, we'll explain the different forms that cannabis can come in, from the plant to all the various manufactured products, and how they might provide different effects.

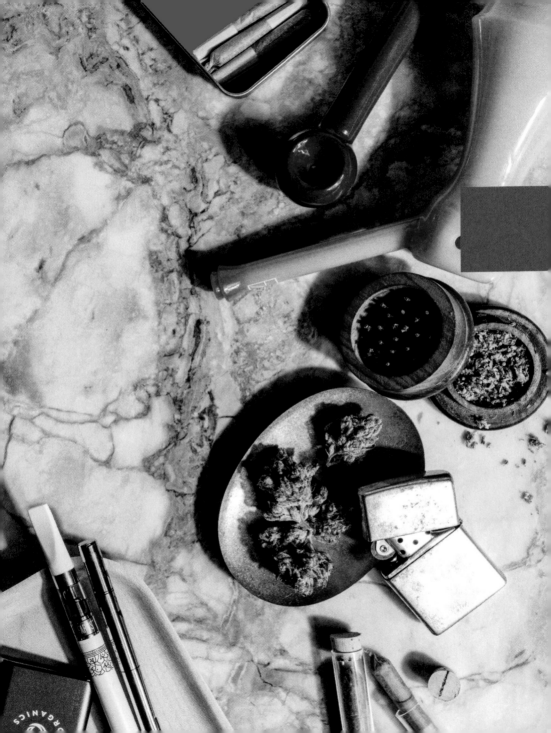

CHAPTER 6

Forms of Cannabis—From Buds to Brownies and Beyond

We've talked about the different compounds within the cannabis plant, including cannabinoids and terpenes, that can nourish our endocannabinoid system (ECS) and promote health and wellness. To understand the various ways of utilizing the plant to get it into our bodies, we should first be able to recognize the different forms cannabis can come in depending on how it is processed and produced.

As cannabis is legalized state by state and the cannabis industry matures, companies are manufacturing a variety of products from the plant. You may see newer forms of processed cannabis for consumption coming onto the market, such as cannabis sublingual breath strips, nasal sprays, and inhalers. The way cannabis is processed can affect the quality, potency (strength of the product), and longevity (shelf life) of the finished product.

FROM SEED TO SALE

Let's look at the how the cannabis plant is processed before it turns into the products you purchase. The processing of cannabis flower from planting seeds to selling it at a licensed cannabis dispensary or retail store—known as "seed to sale"—can take anywhere from five to eight months. Growing the plant can take between three and a half to nearly five months alone, depending on the specific plant being grown as well as how and where it is being grown. Cannabis cultivated indoors will grow and flower more quickly than plants that are grown outdoors. Typically, cannabis grown indoors has a higher THC content than outdoor-grown due to a more controlled, clean environment that isn't at the mercy of Mother Nature.

Cannabis indica takes eight to twelve weeks to be ready to harvest, and *Cannabis sativa* takes ten to sixteen weeks. Growing is the first step to getting cannabis to market. Harvesting the plant is a time-intensive process that happens once the female cannabis plants are mature and have flowered. The way cannabis is grown, treated while growing (such as administering pesticides and plant nutrients), and harvested differs from farm to farm.

In a perfect world, the cannabis you consume would be free of pesticides. However, not all producers take on the expense and complex task of growing pesticide-free plants. Some cannabis products involve extraction processes that can remove pesticide residue. Some states put regulations in place requiring testing for pesticides. Check manufacturer websites to see if they specify their approach to pesticides and testing. In terms of harvesting, some farms use more automation than others, although certain parts of the process—such as trimming the buds to remove stems and leaves—are still handled manually.

The three main steps of harvesting cannabis plants are the following:

1   Removing the large fan leaves from the female plant. These are the larger serrated leaves you recognize as cannabis that are not typically consumed but can be juiced for their nutrient content without any high.

2   Removing what is known as *trim*, which are smaller leaves and stems closer to the flower buds that can be used to produce concentrated oils for topical products or oils and butters for edibles.

3   Picking the flowers and flower buds from the plant stem, which remain on the plant's branches, that are eventually smoked, vaped, or made into more concentrated forms of cannabis.

Once pulled from the plants, the flowers and leaves are sorted, dried, and cured, typically as branches hanging in a drying room. Drying cannabis leaves can take from five to fifteen days. After the cannabis is dried or cured, it is manicured, which involves removing flowers and leaves from branches and then trimming them. Trimmed buds are placed into airtight containers such as glass canning jars, or containers made of metal, plastic, or ceramics. (The key here is that the storage containers are airtight. Gone are the days of storing cannabis in plastic bags that let in oxygen that degrades the quality of the plant matter more quickly.)

The cannabis is stored in a dry, dark place for several weeks to complete the curing process. The dried plant matter is then rehydrated and the containers are opened briefly several times to let the flowers breathe. Extending the curing process four to eight weeks can optimize the final plant product, and some cannabis strains are cured for months. Black-market cannabis tends to be rushed through the harvesting process to get to selling product quickly. You can ask your budtender about growing details when you purchase cannabis flower; however, this is not always information passed on from the grower. Someday, cannabis flower may be marketed like wine, with extensive data on cultivation, curing, and processing for the more discerning consumer.

Legal commercial cannabis cultivators often prefer a longer curing process, like aging a fine wine, while the licensed sellers—the dispensaries—are eager to get product on the shelves, so sometimes the quality of the cannabis you buy is affected by supply and demand. Licensed manufacturers are also in the production chain ready to process the cannabis plant into the different forms of cannabis, which adds more time between harvest and the delivery of actual products to dispensaries and stores. Freshness is important when purchasing cannabis flower but processed cannabis will typically have an extended shelf life.

Picking a quality cannabis product can prove challenging, even when you follow the guidelines outlined in this book. While you can ask friends, family members, or colleagues who consume for their opinions, the feedback you get might be inconsistent or not relevant to your needs. Buying from a trusted dispensary with a good reputation and positive reviews is a good place to start. Work with a knowledgeable medical professional, health practitioner, or cannabis consultant if you can. Visit reputable websites for online product reviews, attend cannabis-related educational events, or read cannabis industry trade publications for information on manufacturers. Knowing what forms of cannabis exist helps you select the right products for your needs.

FORMS OF CANNABIS

Let's break down the different forms of cannabis and discuss how they are processed, starting with the forms closest to the natural state of the plant. Choosing the form of cannabis that is right for you can depend on how you want to consume it and how it works with your body, both of which we will discuss in the next chapter.

FLOWER (BUD)

Cannabis flowers are the hairy, sticky parts of the female plant that are harvested and dried for consumption. Cannabis in its most common and minimally processed form has been called many things in the past: *flower, herb, bud, grass, weed, pot,* and even *leaf* although it is specifically the flower, and not the leaf, that is being referenced. Heat must be applied to dried cannabis flower to activate it and convert the naturally occurring cannabinoid THCA to THC. Therefore, dried cannabis flower is generally smoked or vaped (see pages 75 to 80) to apply heat to the dried plant material.

Typically, at dispensaries or stores, you'll see dried cannabis flower or buds displayed in glass or plastic containers, sometimes with a magnifying glass built into the lid to let you examine the plant matter more closely. Some of the dried plant is also ground and used in pre-rolls or joints (which are like rolled cigarettes) using rolling papers (which could be made of hemp paper or other materials). Depending on local laws, pre-rolls might be rolled in-house at dispensaries or might be manufactured by a company licensed to process and package cannabis.

If you are looking for the benefits of CBD without too much THC, there are strains that tend to be higher in CBD that will temper the THC, such as ACDC with a CBD-to-THC ratio of 20:1, Ringo's Gift at 24:1, Cannatonic with about a 5:1 ratio, and Harlequin with a 5:2 ratio. Ratios in flower are not precise and can vary greatly based on the device you use to consume it, and whether you smoke, vape, or ingest it in some other way.

Kief is a by-product of ground dried cannabis flower and consists of powdery dried trichomes from the plant that often fall through cannabis grinders. Kief can be added to flower that is smoked or vaped to increase its potency. It can also be pressed to create hash or put under additional pressure to make a more concentrated form, rosin (see page 68).

CONCENTRATES

Just as it sounds, concentrates are more concentrated forms of cannabis derived from flower and trim using various types of extraction processes. Manufacturers take the plant matter and treat it to produce forms of cannabis with higher levels of THC and other cannabinoids and terpenes contained within the cannabis plant. CBD-heavy concentrates are processed from strains with higher CBD-to-THC ratios, while some isolate the CBD and eliminate the THC.

Cannabis extraction may use solvents such as butane, propane, carbon dioxide, ethanol, and CO_2 oil, some of which can leave an unhealthful or even toxic residue that may or may not be removed, depending on local laws around testing and the integrity of the manufacturer. There are also solventless extraction methods that are often preferred by more health-conscious consumers, although keep in mind that cannabis is as clean as the grower grows it. Different forms of concentrates include the following.

Butane hash oil (BHO) is a potent, concentrated form of cannabis that is oily and sticky in consistency. *Honeycomb* is BHO that has hardened and become crumbly. *Shatter* is BHO that is more crisp and translucent, like glass. Depending on the plant processed, BHO can contain up to 80 percent THC. However, the butane used to make BHO is toxic. Check for product test results that show the butane has been removed from what you purchase or look for some of the concentrates listed here that don't use toxic solvents. When in doubt, ask your budtender.

CO_2 oil is extracted using pressure and carbon dioxide in a process called supercritical fluid extraction, a solventless method. While effective for extraction, the resulting oil is typically combined with an additive to thin it when used in disposable vape pens and cartridges. Polypropylene glycol is the most common additive, and there are health concerns around inhaling or ingesting this chemical. When heated, polypropylene glycol can turn into formaldehyde. Look for CO2-extracted concentrates that do not use polypropylene glycol by asking specifically for them when visiting a dispensary. A less volatile thinning agent is vegetable glycerin. Newer supercritical extraction technology is also producing thinner oils that might not require thinning agents.

Hash is made from compressing plant resin, or even kief, to produce a more concentrated form of dried cannabis. Hash is typically crumbly or a little sticky but is more of a dry product versus a wet product like oil. It is also considered more old-school as newer forms of concentrates have hit the market. Pressure, not solvents, are used to make hash.

Live resin is a type of cannabis concentrate that is made by flash freezing freshly harvested cannabis and keeping it frozen at subcritical temperatures throughout the extraction process. Live resin is another solventless concentrate.

Rick Simpson oil (RSO) is a highly concentrated form of cannabis oil and, yes, there really is a Rick Simpson. In 2003, he documented his recipe for this oil that he claims cured his skin cancer. The tarlike, oily liquid is produced using naphtha or isopropyl alcohol to extract compounds from the plant. The solvent evaporates once the extraction process is complete.

Rosin is derived through a process of intense heat and pressure that squeezes rosin or sap from plant material, including flowers, hash, and kief. This extraction method does not require solvents. Rosin can actually be made using a flat iron (a two-inch model with a low-heat setting of less than 300°F [149°C] will work best) and parchment paper if you're so inclined. Because rosin is a solventless method of extraction, it is preferred by people who worry about traces of toxic residue.

TINCTURES

Historically, tinctures were the main form of cannabis medicine until cannabis prohibition in the early part of the twentieth century. Tinctures are a liquid form of concentrated cannabis extractions, usually extracted using grain alcohol or a fat-soluble liquid such as glycerol and contained in an alcohol or vegetable-glycerin base stored in glass bottles with droppers used for dosing. The cannabis plant material—flowers or trim—used to make tinctures must be decarboxylated (or heated) first, so using flowers straight from a live plant won't produce the cannabinoids THC or CBD. Decarbing is part of the commercial manufacturing process to make cannabis and CBD tinctures and must be done when making tinctures at home to activate the acid forms of cannabinoids. Today, some "tinctures" use medium-chain triglyceride (MCT) oil as a base, namely coconut oil. Technically, cannabis-infused coconut oil is not a tincture, but it comes in dropper bottles and is often referred to as one.

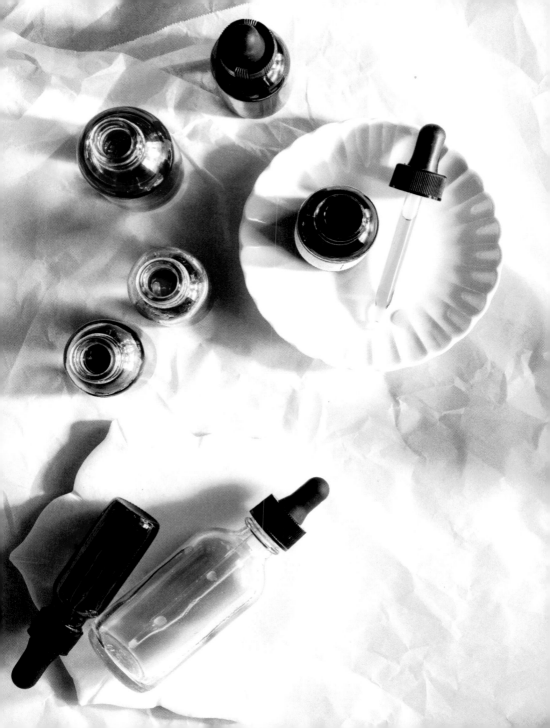

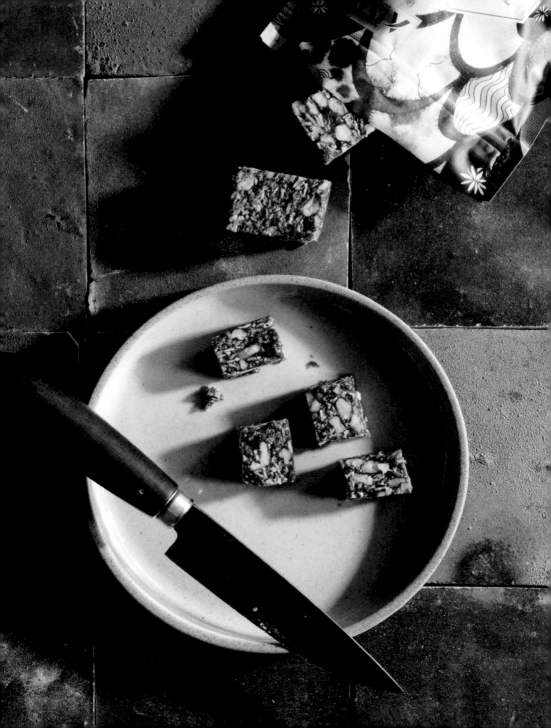

INGESTIBLES INCLUDING EDIBLES

Until markets for cannabis became open and legal, most edible or drinkable forms of cannabis were tinctures, capsules, and foods cooked using cannabis-infused butters or oils. Cannabinoids are fat soluble so infusing fatty butters and oils increases absorption. Consuming decarboxylated cannabis in food and drinks is no longer limited to baked goods and homemade remedies. Today, there are myriad ingestible cannabis products.

Modern-day edibles include candies such as gummies, lollipops, mints, and chocolates; baked goods such as cookies, brownies, and granola; savory foods such as crackers, cheeses, and jerky; and drinkables such as coffee, tea, juice, wine, and water. Other ingestible forms of cannabis taken orally and swallowed include capsules, dissolvable tablets or breath strips, and oral sprays.

As you can see, there is no dearth of cannabis forms for delivery into your system to achieve health and wellness benefits, and new forms are being developed as the cannabis industry continues to mature. For each form of cannabis, there is a delivery method—or several methods—to match. Let's explore those next.

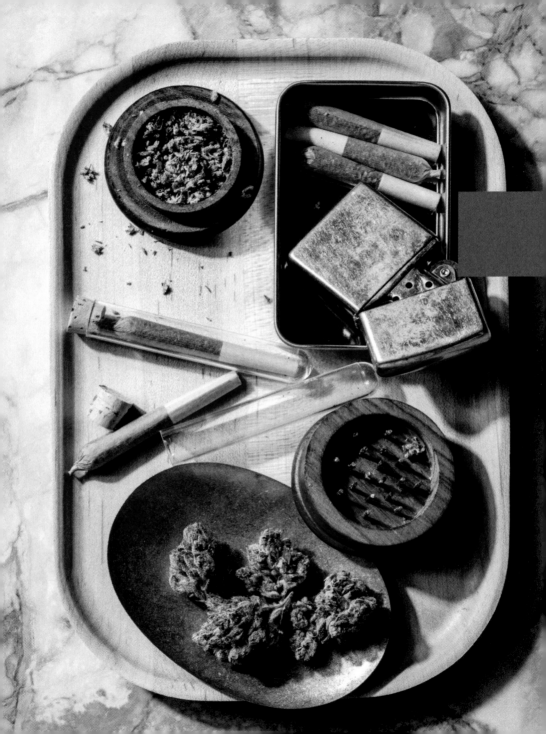

CHAPTER 7

Ways to Take in Cannabis—From Pipes and Bongs to Edibles and Oils

What are the best ways to benefit from the therapeutic properties of cannabis and CBD? How do you deliver the beneficial parts of the plant into your body? Are some ways of consuming better than others? These are all great questions that we'll answer in this chapter.

We've talked about the main forms of cannabis, from the plant's natural state to various forms and products made using different methods of processing. As cannabis becomes legal in more places, companies are developing products that process the cannabis plant matter for you, manufacturing ready-to-use products that are easy to take and tolerate.

The methods for consuming cannabis require processing the plant in some manner before consuming it. While there are differing opinions on which delivery methods are more—or less—healthful, your choices boil down to what effects you're seeking and your personal preferences. Regardless of the form or delivery method you use to get cannabis into your body, the prevailing wisdom is always "start low and go slow." Take small amounts—a few puffs, half a tablet, a fourth of an edible to start—and see how you feel before incrementally increasing the dose over time.

Let's start with the minimally processed form of the plant—raw leaves and dried flower—and work our way through more manufactured products and how to use them. Keep in mind that products with THC are available in the states where they are legal but until cannabis is federally legal, cannabis cannot cross state lines.

RAW CANNABIS LEAVES

Believe it or not, you can juice the fresh, raw leaves of the cannabis plant—the fan leaves—and get therapeutic benefits from them as a dietary supplement without getting high. Why is that? In the raw, untreated cannabis plant, cannabinoids are in their acid form so THC, the psychotropic cannabinoid in cannabis, is still in the form called THCA. Unless the plant matter is dried and heated or burned to decarboxylate it, the compounds within raw cannabis are not mind-altering. Likewise, CBD in raw cannabis leaves is still in its acid form CBGA. (See page 38 for the features and benefits of CBGA.)

Juicing raw cannabis leaves is similar to juicing leafy vegetables. Seek out organically grown plants to reduce the amount of harmful chemicals and pesticides contained within and on the leaves. Raw cannabis leaves taste slightly bitter, spicy, and earthy with the pungent flavor of cannabis. While it can be an acquired taste, you can also cut the flavor by adding other fruit or vegetable juices. The raw leaves contain vitamins, minerals, and amino acids, in addition to the acid forms of cannabinoids including THCA, CBDA, and CBGA. Juicing cannabis leaves can provide your body with antioxidant, anti-inflammatory, and immune-boosting effects. While technically you cannot buy raw cannabis leaves commercially, you can obtain raw cannabis leaves by purchasing a cannabis clone and growing your own plant.

INHALATION

Inhaling cannabis can mean either burning or heating the dried plant to convert it into a form that your body can absorb. Before inhaling dried cannabis, you might grind the dry buds of the plant to roll a joint for smoking. You might warm dried, ground cannabis flower in a personal vaporizer or vape pen to decarboxylate, or activate, the THC. Let's look at smoking and vaping more closely.

SMOKING

Smoking cannabis is similar to smoking a cigarette or pipe. You suck on a device or tool that burns the plant matter and allows you to bring the smoke into your lungs. While some people hold in cannabis smoke, there isn't really a need to do this as the smoke will enter your lungs and be absorbed immediately. Holding the smoke in your lungs doesn't get you higher because you are taking in the same amount of smoke with each inhale. Holding in smoke is most likely going to get you a little dizzy from lack of oxygen, and holding it in too long can cause bronchial irritation and coughing. Some common tools used for burning dry cannabis flower to smoke it are as follows.

Joints are made with ground dried cannabis flower wrapped in paper that can be in a cylinder or cone shape. These are also referred to as *pre-rolls* or *cannabis cigarettes*, blunts (rolled in cigar paper), or spliffs (mixed with tobacco). California-based Herbabuena's whole-flower pre-rolled joints are available in CBD flower as well as sativa and indica versions. Smoking a joint is similar to smoking a cigarette. You can hold it to your lips and light it with a match or lighter as you suck in, but some people prefer using a hemp wick (available at smoke shops and dispensaries) that is lit first and held to a joint or other smoking device for a less toxic light (without sulfur or butane). You can also opt for an electric lighter that does not use butane. Some people use cigarette holders or joint tips made of paper or even glass to protect their fingers and lips as the joint burns down. A metal clip, also called a roach clip, is an old-school method of holding a joint using a clip to keep the burning material away from your fingers.

Pipes come in many shapes and sizes, from *spoons* (standard bowl and stem) and *steamrollers* (cylinders with a chamber) to *one-hitters* (cigarette-shaped pipes for one hit or dose of cannabis flower). Pipes can be simple and plain or elaborately embellished, making for real conversation pieces. They are made from nonflammable materials such as metal, glass, hardwood, stone, ceramic, or silicone. Some pipes have a *carb,* or small hole that helps clear the chamber. To use a carb, hold your thumb over the hole and release it as you are finishing inhaling to propel the smoke into your lungs rapidly and deeply. You can purchase pipes legally (if you are twenty-one or older) at smoke shops, dispensaries, online head shops such as DankStop, or directly from companies that manufacture specialty models, such as Jane West.

Water pipes or bongs are devices that include a body chamber that holds water, a stem with a bowl at one end to hold and burn dried cannabis, and a mouthpiece or opening, usually at the end of a tube. To use one, seal the tube over your mouth and inhale, drawing smoke from the bowl through the stem and water, and up through the body chamber and tube into your mouth and lungs. There is also a carb on the body of the bong that is used like a carb on a cannabis pipe with similar results. You can usually find bongs for purchase in the same places you find pipes: smoke shops, dispensaries, and online head shops as well as through specialty bong makers such as My Bud Vase.

VAPING

Vaporizing, or vaping, cannabis can be a fast delivery method of either dried cannabis or cannabis and CBD concentrates using a battery- or electricity-operated device called a vaporizer or vape pen. Some popular flower or loose-leaf vape pens include the Pax 2 from Pax, and IQ and MicroIQ from DaVinci. Dried, finely ground cannabis is placed in an internal chamber within the vaporizer. If you're vaping oil, it usually comes in a removable cartridge that you attach to an oil vaporizer or it could come ready-to-vape in a disposable vape pen. While some vaporizers can handle both dried flower and oil, most are designed for one or the other. The Pax 3, for example, accommodates both cannabis flower and extracts, while the Pax Era is for oils only that are contained in square pods, designed by the Pax company, instead of the more common round cartridges.

A vaporizer or vape pen is battery run—either disposable or rechargeable—and turned on (usually with five clicks) to warm the cannabis at either low, medium, or high temperatures set by the manufacturer or a manual control. Vapor is produced by the warming action, releasing cannabinoids and terpenes from the cannabis.

Vaping temperatures are lower than burning temps, usually under 455°F (235°C). Some vape pens offer a feature that gives you more control over the temperature settings to release different cannabinoids and terpenes at different temperatures. For many people, vaping feels less harsh and irritating than smoking cannabis.

Vaping devices come in many sizes, from tabletop vaporizers and handheld vape pens to cartridge, or "cart," batteries that connect with oil cartridges. Handheld models can be small enough to hold in one hand or even nestle into your palm so you can close your fingers around it for discreet vaping, such as the Ario Vape Contour line of cart batteries. You can buy cylinder, or "stick," and other shaped cartridge batteries at smoke shops, dispensaries, and online head shops and use them by twisting standard oil cartridges onto them.

You can also purchase disposable vape pens, cylindrically shaped like cigarettes, that warm concentrated cannabis oil stored inside when you draw on the mouthpiece and inhale. Good disposable vape pen manufacturers include Select CBD (CBD and terpenes only), Lucid Mood, Mozen, Dosist, and Wildflower, just to name a few. Some companies, such as Wildflower, also make cartridges in addition to disposable pens. The company Bloom Farms manufactures disposable vape pens, standard cartridges, and Pax-specific cartridges. Unloaded vape pens can be purchased in the same places as pipes and bongs. Preloaded, disposable vape pens and oil cartridges can only be obtained through dispensaries unless they contain hemp-derived CBD with no THC.

The chart below can be used as a guide to the cannabinoids and terpenes released at various temperatures. If you have a vape pen with temperature controls, set it according to the cannabinoid or terpene you'd like released, but keep in mind the cannabis product you purchase should test positive for that particular compound.

Boiling Points of Cannabis Compounds

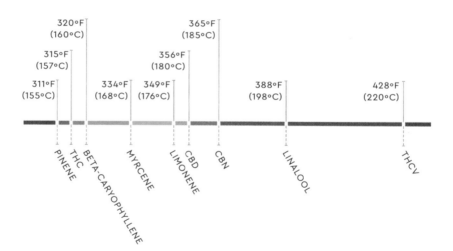

DABBING

A more potent form of vaporizing cannabis concentrates is called *dabbing*. To dab, you need a *dab rig*, or vaping device that includes a heating element, or *nail*, usually made of titanium to withstand high heat. The nail is heated with a powerful heat source, like a butane torch. When a concentrated form of cannabis, typically a more solid form such as shatter, wax, budder, or crumble, is placed on the hot nail, it immediately vaporizes. That vapor is directed through the dab rig and mouthpiece into your mouth and then lungs as you inhale. The effects of dabbing are fast and very strong. Dabbing is ideal for people with acute pain or conditions that require stronger medicine. Dabbing is also popular with individuals looking to get very high very quickly for recreational purposes. Try to only dab pure concentrates extracted without any chemicals (solventless) to take in a clean vapor. Dab rigs are available at most smoke shops, online head shops, and some dispensaries.

INHALERS

Breathing in a cannabis concentrated liquid formula as a mist through an inhaler is another way of consuming cannabis with fast results. Cannabis inhalers are most commonly used either for medicinal intake or as a healthier alternative to smoking, vaping, or dabbing. Typical cannabis inhalers contain about 1000 milligrams of liquid, which accounts for about 100 puffs at about 10 milligrams per puff. Some cannabis inhalers on the market include Santana Smooth by Marisol Therapeutics and the Aerohalter from the Revered Company.

INGESTION

From cookies, brownies, candies, and other sweets to savory, salty, and spicy food items, today's medicated edible food products are as varied as food itself. Virtually any type of food can be infused with cannabis, although fatty foods are best because cannabis is fat soluble, and new food items are hitting the shelves every month. Some popular cannabis-infused edibles include cannabis gummies from Wana and CBD gummies from Lord and Jones, chocolate by Kiva Confections, and raw cacao from Whoopi & Maya. How about something savory, like a tomato-basil soup mix from American Baked Company or cheese biscuits from Auntie Delores? The edibles choices are seemingly endless.

Wanting more of a cannabis or CBD culinary experience? You'll find events in some legal states offering medicated meals where chefs produce multiple courses with CBD and cannabis-infused dishes, such as the ones produced by Chef Matt in California. He caters events, including weddings, and offers personal chef services.

Ready-to-drink beverages are available on the market and don't require special equipment to ingest, and include CBD-infused bottled water such as CBD Living Water and cannabis-infused coffee from Somatik, sodas such as California Dreamin' and Sprig, specialty drinks such as GT's Kombucha, energy drinks such as Lifted by Dixie Elixirs, and even beer such as Ceria from the founder of Blue Moon or Two Roots Brewing Company, and wine from Rebel Coast Winery and Saka Wines. You can also find infused ground coffee such as Steepfuze or loose or bagged tea that you can prepare at home from Kikoko or Stillwater. Even Coca-Cola announced in 2018 that they were looking into producing a CBD-infused beverage.

While some food or drink edibles might have a distinct cannabis flavor, many are using new technologies to infuse without a strong taste or aftertaste. Edibles do not provide an instant effect because once you swallow them, they take time to go through your entire digestive system and get processed by your liver. Time of onset, or when effects are felt from edibles or any method of delivery, differs for each person because of many variables, including metabolism. The effects of edibles can last longer than other forms of consumption because of how it is processed in your body. Your liver alters the cannabinoid content of the cannabis you've ingested, including converting the form of THC that is absorbed into your bloodstream, making it potentially more potent than other forms.

CAPSULES AND TABLETS

If you are looking for less taste in your mouth or a more controlled dose with a time-released effect, capsules or tablets might be an option for you. More companies are manufacturing what amounts to pharmaceutical-style capsules and pills that you can purchase based on dosage amounts and take orally with water or any other liquid (although we wouldn't recommend taking with alcohol because it could alter or lessen the beneficial effects of cannabis). Like edibles, capsules or tablets that you swallow whole will take time to produce the effects, which can last a few hours. Capsules and tablets are easy to carry and discreet with no telltale odor or mess. Look for products from companies such as Dr. Robb Farms, including their Mom's Formula line (tablets—and not just for women); Equilibria (CBD capsules); and Altus (tablets).

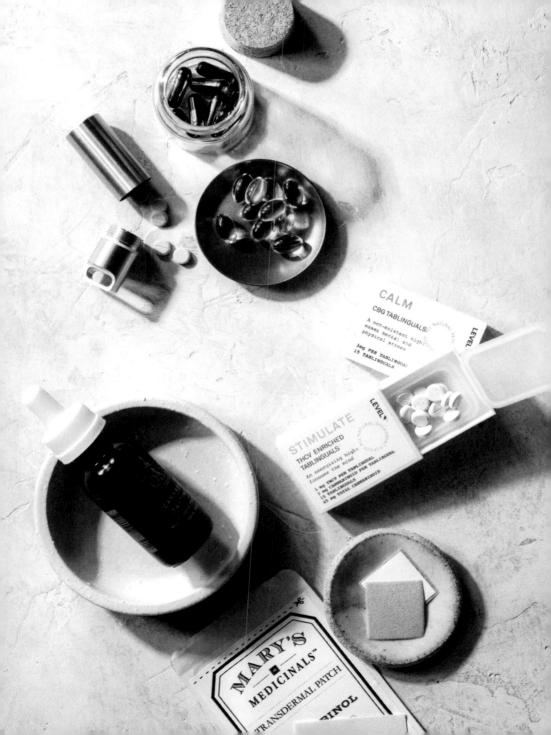

TINCTURES

Although all of the mucous membranes of your mouth can absorb tinctures effectively, drops are usually placed under the tongue for fast absorption. You'll feel the effects of a tincture containing THC more rapidly than edibles and pills. Alcohol-based tinctures may sting the mucous membranes under your tongue but are less likely to burn when swished around your entire mouth before swallowing. Today, some "tinctures" use medium-chain triglyceride oil (MCT), namely coconut oil. Technically, cannabis-infused coconut oil is not a tincture, but it can be found in dropper bottles and most people call them tinctures anyway. One advantage of an MCT-based tincture is that it is less harsh on your mouth's mucous membranes so it doesn't sting when you use it. Another advantage of an oil-based oral tincture is that cannabinoids are stored in fat, not water; since cannabinoids are fat-soluble, this makes the cannabis extracts more easily absorbed into your body. While consuming cannabis with fat increases absorption; placing drops into other, nonfatty liquids such as coffee, tea, juice, or water can slow absorption.

You can make a tincture with a jar, alcohol, and a strainer. You can find recipes for alcohol- and oil-based tinctures on websites or in books such as *A Woman's Guide to Cannabis* by Nikki Furrer. Tinctures are kept in glass bottles so be careful that they don't break, leak, or spill—carry them with care. They may also have an odor so you will want to keep the bottle in a sealable, waterproof, odor-resistant bag. Tinctures can be a good form for dosing in increments although they are not as precise as tablets. Some popular tincture companies include ONDA Wellness CBD, the Alchemist's Kitchen, and CBDAlive, which are CBD specific. Good CBD and THC tinctures can be purchased from Juna, Papa & Barkley, and Care by Design.

WATER-SOLUBLE POWDER

Water-soluble powder can be dissolved quickly and easily into any liquid (including water, coffee, tea, juice, soda), mixtures such as pasta sauce or applesauce, and foods such as yogurt and pudding. Water-soluble powders, like the ones produced by Stillwater, come in packets similar to artificial sweeteners and can contain THC, CBD, and other cannabinoids depending on the manufacturing process. These powders provide effects similar to manufactured edibles but give you more control over the dose and are especially handy for microdosing (which is covered in chapter 8). The technology that produces this type of powder requires isolating the cannabinoids so they are essentially isolates and not whole-plant extracts. Depending on the product you purchase, powders can come in different ratios of CBD to THC or contain only CBD. Odorless, portable, discreet, and flavorless are some features of water-soluble powders.

ORAL ABSORPTION

Other than tinctures, products for oral absorption include sprays, like Life Bloom Organics' Wellness or Sleep CBD formulas; sublingual (under the tongue) tablets from Level; and dissolvable strips, similar to breath strips like those from Kin Slips. Sprays are usually dosed between 1 and 5 milligrams per spray and can be applied under the tongue, on the tongue, or anywhere in the mouth and swallowed. Sublingual tablets are held under the tongue until they dissolve and are then swallowed. Dissolvable strips are placed on the tongue and dissolve quickly. As with tinctures, oral absorption products enter your bloodstream quickly, including through your sublingual glands, and can last a few hours.

Some oral cannabis products, particularly CBD-only ones, tout using nanotechnology to manipulate cannabis molecules at the anatomic level to increase absorption. While this claim of rapid absorption may be accurate, there are no studies yet that prove nano-based products are good or bad for you. Because the wisdom on consumption is "start low, go slow," the jury is still out on chemically manipulating cannabis molecules to enter your bloodstream even faster than they would in a less altered form. Sprays, tablets, and breath strips can be more measurable and are portable, discreet, and virtually odor-free.

NASAL ABSORPTION

Mucous membranes of the mouth aren't the only area on your body that are more permeable and facilitate the absorption of liquid-based cannabis. Like oral sprays, nasal mists, as those produced by Verra Wellness, are a fast-acting, discreet method of consumption. Simply insert the nozzle into your nostril and spray gently, no need to inhale.

TOPICALS

Cannabis-infused or CBD-containing topicals are products that you apply to the surface of your skin, and depending on how they are made and where on the body you use them, they can have different absorption rates and benefits. Topicals are typically infused with concentrated forms of cannabis or isolated forms of THC, CBD, or other cannabinoids and terpenes developed through standard extraction processes.

Topicals containing THC, like Papa & Barkley Releaf Balm and Whoopi & Maya's Rub, are exclusively available at licensed dispensaries. Topicals with CBD only that are derived from industrial hemp may be found at mainstream retailers, from drug stores to health food stores to salons and spas, depending on where you live, although most of the mainstream stores carry hemp products that don't contain CBD. Other products from companies such as Dr. Kerklaan, Apothecanna, and CBDistillery sell online and ship throughout the United States. (In some states or cities, CBD may still be regulated or banned despite the 2019 Farm Bill.) Products made with CBD derived from the same plant as THC versus industrial hemp–derived ones may be regulated similarly to cannabis and carried in dispensaries, depending on where you live.

Some products you might see on the market for topical application include the following:

- Bath bombs
- Creams
- Lip balms
- Lotions
- Oils
- Ointments
- Roll-ons (solid and liquid)
- Salves
- Sprays
- Transdermal patches

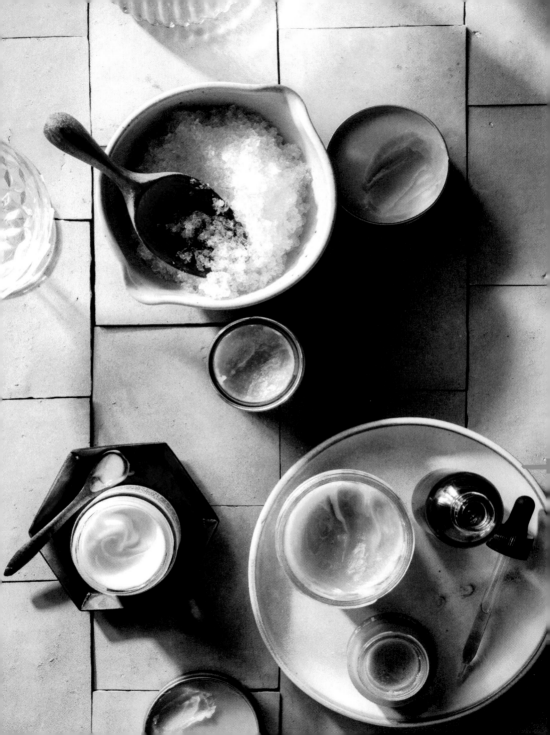

As with any cannabis or CBD product, ask a budtender, manager, or customer service rep at a dispensary or retailer for recommendations; review manufacturer websites; contact the company for product features; and read reviews and ratings online from trusted sources. Also, read the labels for all the ingredients contained in the topical to make sure you aren't sensitive or allergic to them, as you would with anything you apply to your skin.

Topicals are nonintoxicating because surface application to your skin usually does not cross the barrier that keeps most topicals from entering your bloodstream or the blood-brain barrier that protects your brain. While a topical that doesn't break these barriers should not show up in a blood or urine test, always use caution when utilizing any cannabis-derived product as there is never a complete guarantee that you will not test positive for cannabis. If you have a cut or open sore on your skin, a topical might enter your bloodstream even if it normally wouldn't.

Some topicals can be made with a penetrating carrier substance—an active pharmaceutical ingredient (API)—that helps the product absorb beneath skin layers and enter your bloodstream. APIs can be liposomes, fatty acids, and even some terpenes (like limonene, linalool, and geraniol) that promote deeper absorption. Oleic acid and emu oil are commonly used in cannabis transdermal products. When purchasing a topical for deeper muscular or joint relief, look for one of the additives we mention or for the term *transdermal* on the label. Any transdermal topicals that affix to your skin, including transdermal patches like the ones from Mary's Medicinals, are most effective when applied to an area of the body with the most veins at the surface, such as your inner wrist, ankles, or neck. Caution: Once the cannabinoids and terpenes in cannabis topicals penetrate into your bloodstream, you could test positive if you are drug tested.

Cannabis topicals or hemp-derived CBD topicals that do not deeply penetrate your skin can be effective to promote healing in inflammation that presents as redness, flakiness, extreme dryness, or rashes; sores or eruptions such as rosacea, psoriasis, and eczema; and acne as well as scrapes and cuts, burns, and even scars. Topicals may also be used for minor muscle and joint pain.

Some benefits of using topicals include addressing either skin irritations or muscular or joint pain in an area-specific manner, giving you the benefits of cannabinoids and sometimes terpenes (if they are contained within the product you're using) without any head high. Topicals can be portable and discreet although some may need to be stored in a cool, dry environment as they may not be as shelf-stable as others.

INSERTION

Another less-talked-about delivery method for cannabis is via suppositories, including vaginal suppositories, such as products by Foria, and rectal suppositories, such as ones sold by Endoca. The vaginal and rectum walls are permeable, like our mouths, so absorption is rapid and effectively targets the lower region of the body. Cannabis suppositories, like any suppositories, are made with dissolvable materials such as gelatin capsules or ingredients like cocoa butter.

Vaginal suppositories dissolve and absorb to provide pain relief and promote body relaxation without mind-altering effects. Vaginal suppositories can be used in relieving pain and inflammation throughout the reproductive system, including the uterus, and for reducing menstrual cramps and pelvic pain from conditions such as polycystic ovary syndrome. THC-infused tampons are also available on the market and can provide relief from menstrual cramps. As with any tampons, changing them regularly is important to avoid health issues such as toxic shock syndrome (TSS). There are no studies or reports stating that THC-infused tampons are any more or less likely to cause TSS. Most cannabis and CBD vaginal products are available at licensed dispensaries although hemp-derived CBD products could be carried at more mainstream retailers.

Rectal suppositories can deliver medicine quickly to relieve pain from irritable bowel syndrome, colitis, Crohn's disease, and other digestive and intestinal discomfort, pain, and disorders. Suppositories are moderately fast-acting—taking twenty to thirty minutes to have an effect—and last anywhere from an hour to a few hours, depending on the strength and all the normal variables from individual to individual.

Now that you're more familiar with the different forms of cannabis and the many different ways you can take cannabis into your body, we're going to go over how to dose cannabis for optimal effects and introduce you to the concept of *microdosing* to get more health benefits with less of the high.

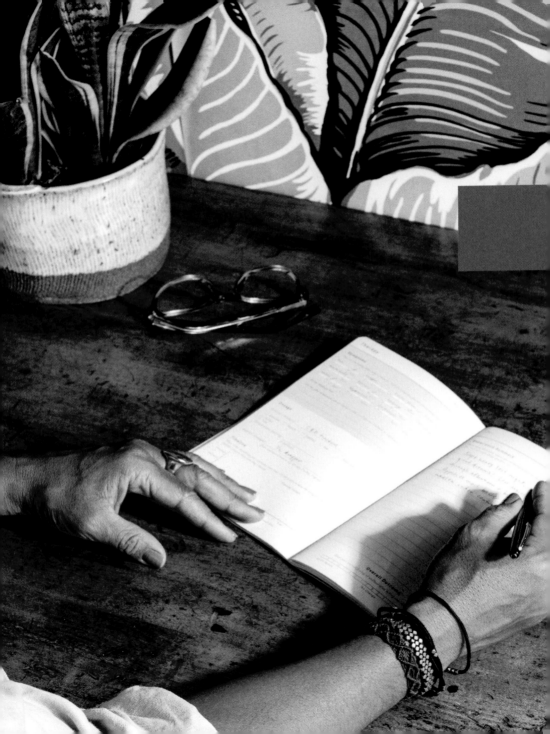

CHAPTER 8

Microdosing THC and CBD

Becoming more familiar with the different forms and delivery methods of cannabis is one thing. Figuring out dosing is another matter entirely. When you take too much cannabis, particularly the cannabinoid THC, you experience mind-altering effects. Many people who are seeking out the health and wellness benefits don't necessarily want to get high. So how can you take nourishing cannabinoids—including the psychotropic THC—into your body without your mind being altered? Enter microdosing.

Microdosing is a moderated consumption method attributed to a Swiss scientist named Dr. Albert Hofmann who, in the 1970s, regularly ingested small doses, or hits, of lysergic acid, better known as LSD. He set out to prove that in smaller doses, a substance with powerful, mind-altering effects could instead provide therapeutic value without the high. He extolled the virtue of a seemingly counterintuitive approach to drug taking, and reported benefits including an overall sense of well-being.

The concept of ingesting smaller doses can apply to cannabis. Microdosing cannabis means consuming low doses of THC repeatedly over a period of time. Low doses of THC can be part of a regular health routine to manage stress, anxiety, and other conditions and disorders. Add CBD into the mix, and you have additional benefits from this popular cannabinoid while also tempering the effects of the THC. You usually would not microdose CBD because its effects are subtler and could take longer to build up in your system before you feel them. Often people say they don't realize CBD is working until they stop taking it and their anxiety, inflammation, or pain returns.

How much THC is considered a microdose? The exact level of THC that constitutes a microdose is relative to the person consuming. A typical microdose is somewhere between 1 and 10 milligrams. Your metabolism, sensitivity to medications, tolerance level, and even what and how much you've had to eat or drink affects how much you should consume and how it will make you feel. If you are sensitive to the effects of THC or are new to cannabis, 2.5 milligrams of THC might be sufficient. If you're more tolerant, particularly if you've been consuming for a longer period of time, 15 milligrams may be more effective for you and still be considered a microdose.

No matter how you consume cannabis or what form you consume, starting low and going slow is the best approach. The same goes for microdosing—start even lower than you'd consider a low dose, then take more incrementally over the course of several days (not all in the same day). When you pass from feeling better to feeling woozy or high, taper back to find your optimal microdose. Have a CBD-only tincture on hand in case you start to feel uncomfortably high. A dose as directed on a bottle of CBD tincture held under your tongue can reduce the high quickly and safely. If you do not have a CBD tincture, chewing on a few peppercorns will also help offset the psychotropic effects of the THC.

SHOULD YOU MICRODOSE?

Microdosing is for anyone who wants to reap the benefits of consuming cannabis without the mind-altering, euphoric, or lethargic effects that come with higher doses of THC. Some people microdose cannabis to stimulate productivity, creativity, and focus.

Before you get started with microdosing, first determine your goal for taking small amounts of THC throughout the day. The most common reasons to microdose are to reduce anxiety and inflammation, or to take the edge off of chronic, but not debilitating, pain. Microdoses can be used to help with focus, productivity, and creativity, or even to ease into sleep. However, most people who microdose are addressing a chronic health problem that makes getting through the day a challenge.

Do not consume cannabis if you are taking medications until you've researched all potential interactions, or in medial lingo, make sure cannabis is not contraindicated with any medicine you're currently taking. Do not discontinue any medications you are currently taking in favor of cannabis without trusted, professional guidance, preferably from a physician or naturopath who is knowledgeable about cannabis.

GETTING STARTED WITH MICRODOSING

Zeroing in on what health issue you want to address through microdosing can help you pick the right form of cannabis and method of consumption—either absorbing it orally, ingesting it, smoking, or vaping. Visit your local dispensary to purchase what you need, or if you are in a city and state where cannabis delivery is legal, place an order for products and receive them at your home. California, in particular, offers cannabis delivery through companies such as Eaze, Sava, and Goddess Delivers. For hemp-derived CBD products, find a local store that carries them or order them online for delivery where legal. The websites of reputable companies will specify where they can legally ship.

Before consuming cannabis, particularly for the first time, let at least one trusted friend or family member know what you are planning to do. While consuming cannabis or CBD in the safe environment of your home, particularly in microdoses, is not dangerous, having someone as a backup to look out for you is sensible. Deciding when to take your microdoses depends on your schedule and lifestyle. Start on a weekend when you won't need to drive to work—which can be dangerous under the influence—or ride public transportation, which can be uncomfortable if you take a little too much and experience a high or feel nauseous or dizzy.

Look for information about the potency, recommended doses, and duration of effects on the product packaging or label, get details from a budtender, or locate on the manufacturer's website. Take all product information into consideration before consuming anything. Set reminders on your smartphone to take your microdose at regular intervals throughout the day. Over time, you'll learn how much to take, and when, in order to produce the effects you're seeking.

GETTING THE RIGHT MICRODOSE

Edibles are a common form of cannabis that can be divided into microdosed amounts; however, cannabis-infused foods and drinks are challenging to dose precisely. You can purchase edibles that are already sized for dosing but usually at 5 or 10 milligrams. While you can cut a 10-milligram cookie or chocolate into halves or quarters, there will be some variability to each piece.

A better option for microdosing is a tincture with a dropper. Most cannabis tinctures, especially if not produced for medical use, come with unmarked droppers. You can purchase a dropper or plastic syringe with milligram markings to measure a more accurate dose. Getting accurate doses from tinctures is reliant on the manufacturing company getting their product properly tested for consistency of overall doses of THC or any other cannabinoid contained within the concentrated liquid or oil. Look for products with dosing instructions on the label or information about the strength of each dropperful, then do the math to reduce the content of the dropper to the amount of your ideal dose.

The most reliable way to get a precise dose of THC or other cannabinoids is to take it in pill, capsule, or tablet form from a manufacturer operating with more of a pharmaceutical process. The pills, capsules, and tablets found at cannabis dispensaries should have ingredient and dosing information on their product packaging or label or on their website. Some manufacturers produce tablets and dissolvable tabs in doses as low as 2.5 milligrams, something you're less likely to find in edibles. Candy edibles such as gummies and mints are often dosed around 5 milligrams each. Cutting those in half can give you approximately 2.5 milligrams in each piece. But again, there will be variability.

You can also microdose by smoking or vaping cannabis; however, the doses are much more difficult to measure precisely. While you can't accurately say that one inhale is exactly 5 milligrams, you might, for example, observe that after one inhale you feel relaxed, after two you feel deeply relaxed, and after three you feel sleepy. So if you are microdosing, one or two inhales may be sufficient for you.

It's easy to miss the mark on your ideal dose when inhaling cannabis, so simply taking in a little at a time and gradually increasing until you get the effects you want without the ones you don't is a great way to get started. To feel relaxed or less anxious, or for more focus, you might use a smaller dose. If you'd like help sleeping, you might use a slightly higher dose. Remember that inhaling cannabis produces near-immediate effects while edibles will take a while to go through your system before you feel them. Tinctures and oral sprays or sublinguals will affect you more quickly as well.

DOSING GUIDELINES

The guidelines below start with microdosing and also explain how to incrementally increase or decrease—or *titrate*—both CBD and THC. These are not individualized instructions but general, common techniques. The following process is in no way a personalized medical recommendation for you but simply a framework that explains how microdosing—and regular dosing—are typically handled.

1 Determine the type of delivery system. Typically, you will want to choose one method for immediate relief and another for longer-term relief. For chronic conditions, long-acting oral preparations are the mainstay of treatment. Vaporizing, inhaling, and topical applications are for breakthrough and acute symptoms.

2 Pick your ratio. You can obtain CBD-rich medicine, THC-rich medicine, or a more equal ratio of cannabinoids. A common process is to try ratios in this order: 20:1 CBD-rich medicine, 1:1 CBD/THC balanced, 1:6 THC, 1:20 THC.

3 Pick your product(s). Ask experts such as your budtender or a cannabis consultant, check manufacturer websites, and read reviews from trusted sources. Ask friends or colleagues for anecdotal information but don't rely on nonexperts for definitive advice.

4 Start low and slow with microdosing and titration.

For CBD dosing, begin with a CBD remedy of 15 to 20 milligrams two to three times daily. This can be titrated upward relatively quickly, 5 milligrams at a time, every seven days. With medical guidance, the titration timeframe can be accelerated. Look out for symptoms of stomach upset and diarrhea or worsening versus improving symptoms.

Add THC, if needed, and titrate slowly up. (See the following paragraph for a THC titration framework.) Start with 1 milligram and add 0.5 milligrams every three days until symptom relief, carefully watching out for unwanted side effects, like dizziness or anxiety. Try reaching your optimal therapeutic dosage by adjusting up or down in small increments of CBD and THC. If it's still not working the way you'd like, try a different product.

If no significant improvement is seen in eight weeks, consult a cannabinoid specialist for further adjustments.

For THC dosing, on days one through seven, start with 1 milligram THC before bedtime in case you experience drowsiness as a side effect. On days eight through fourteen, if the previous dose was well tolerated but there is still no symptom relief, increase by increments of 0.5 milligrams THC at bedtime. On days fifteen and on, continue to increase by 0.5 milligrams THC at bedtime as needed. If you experience no adverse effects, you can try to use small amounts of THC during the day until relief is obtained.

You typically will want to take an effective dose every six hours. The goal is to find your optimal therapeutic dose without experiencing unwanted side effects.

If you are using THC, be careful not to operate machinery or anything that requires balance and dexterity or fast reflexes as THC may alter your perception. Do not drive while under the influence of THC.

TRACKING YOUR MICRODOSING

Until cannabis becomes federally legal and is produced with proper and consistent testing and manufactured in precisely measured doses, microdosing should begin with the lowest doses, incrementally increasing, and monitoring the outcomes each step of the way. Keep a journal of your process. You can do this with an old-fashioned notebook and pen, or download a cannabis journal or tracking app to keep track of what you take.

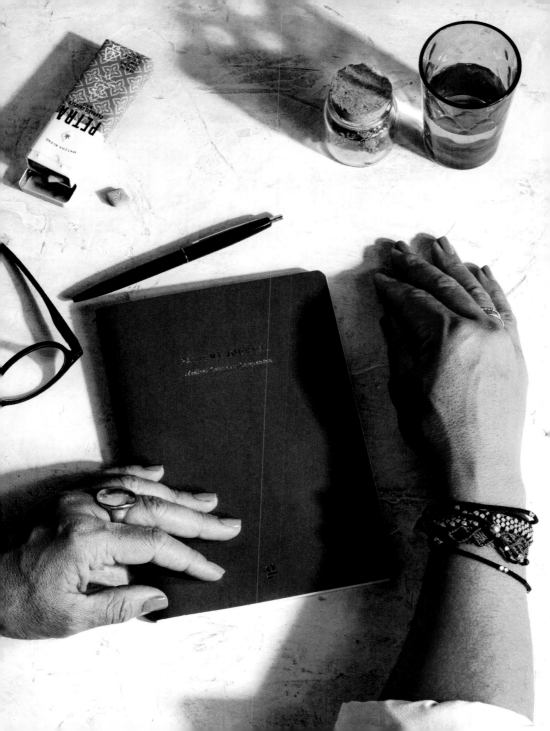

Here are some observations you should record in a THC or CBD journal:

- ▶ Date and time
- ▶ Goal(s)
- ▶ Product(s) taken (strains, ratios, dominant ingredients, whatever is known)
- ▶ Dose(s) taken
- ▶ Time(s) taken
- ▶ Onset of effects (how long before you felt them)
- ▶ Effects (what kind and specify from mild to strong)
- ▶ Duration in minutes/hours
- ▶ Other medications or supplements taken and when
- ▶ Meals and snacks eaten and when
- ▶ Feelings before dosing (and specify from mild to strong)
- ▶ Feelings after dosing
- ▶ Outcome (worse, no change, better, optimal)

Record the time of day you ingest, note what you've had to eat or drink, and your mood before and after consumption, and detail the effects you feel—both positive and negative—including how long they last. Track the THC and CBD ratios of the products you consume as well as the strains, if you know them. Remember that CBD can temper THC so is often helpful when you have both in the cannabis products you consume.

Reputable dispensaries will clearly identify cannabis strains and provide you with a printout of test results that outline the percentages of each main compound contained in the product. State-regulated cannabis products will contain details on the packaging, often depending on the laws for the location where they are produced and sold. Most manufacturers include testing results on their websites. If you can't easily obtain testing results for manufactured products, look for alternatives products from companies that are willing and able to disclose this critical information.

Over time, you should be able to determine not only what form of cannabis works best for you but also how to measure a proper dose for what you consume. If you're new to cannabis or previously had an unpleasant experience with it, microdosing can be a more comfortable introduction or reintroduction to the benefits of the plant without dealing with extreme effects.

If you're looking for incremental relief or effects over time, microdosing is ideal. If you're experiencing more acute conditions that require stronger medicine, cannabis can also be used in that manner.

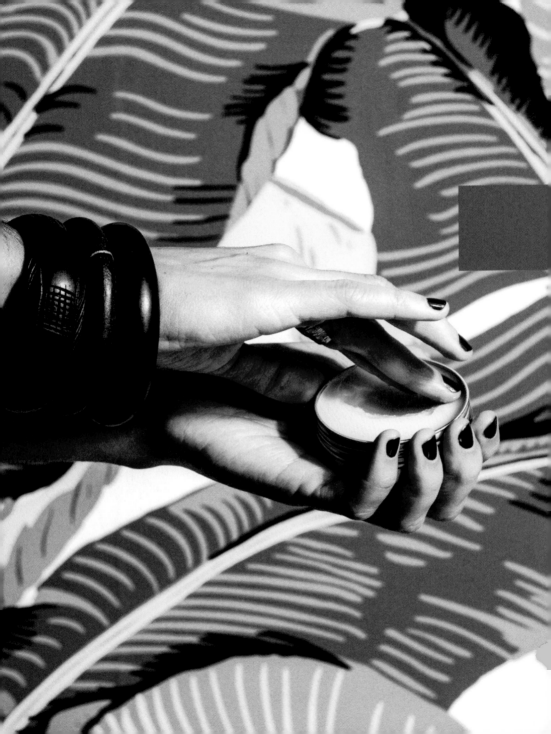

CHAPTER 9

Cannabis and Acute Conditions

Throughout this book, we've mentioned a variety of conditions that can be treated using cannabis and its derivatives. Now let's delve a little more deeply into some common acute conditions and how cannabis can help. We've included stories from actual patients of Dr. Chin's to illustrate real-life applications of cannabis for acute conditions.

Note that these anecdotes are meant to illustrate how cannabis can be used therapeutically and are not meant as individual recommendations for you or someone you know. At the end of each story, we include a short list of cannabinoids and terpenes that can address the specific issues mentioned, but they are not medical recommendations and do not address any underlying conditions.

CONDITION: NAUSEA

Harold was a thin, frail-looking man who came into Dr. Chin's office complaining of chronic nausea and acid reflux. After years as a sickly child unable to properly eat, digest, or absorb nutrients from his food, in college he discovered that cannabis before a meal relieved some of his symptoms, and he could eat without nausea. Years later, extensive testing with a specialist at Mayo Clinic finally revealed a diagnosis: gastroparesis, a chronic condition with symptoms including vomiting, nausea, acid reflux, and abdominal bloating and pain.

> "The fullness and tightness in my stomach began to disappear, and I felt less gas pains."

The human brain has nausea and vomiting trigger centers. These brain centers have receptors that also control the digestive tract. Antinausea pharmaceutical medications, like ondansetron and prochlorperazine, work on these receptor centers in the brain. So does cannabis. The side effects of pharmaceutical medications are often constipation and the slowing down of the digestive system. A patient with gastropareisis cannot afford to put the brakes on an already slow-moving digestive tract.

For Harold, Dr. Chin recommended a CBD-dominant sublingual tincture ratio of 20 CBD to 1 THC rich in limonene. Harold began using the 20:1 tincture at a low starting dose of 15 milligrams after breakfast and lunch. He kept track of his dosage and symptoms in a journal. Every seven days, he titrated his dose up by increments of 5 milligrams until he felt an improvement in his bloating, digestion, and stomach pain. When Harold reached 25 milligrams two times a day, he began to feel his bloating and digestion improve.

Unfortunately, Harold did not feel any improvement in nausea and appetite until Dr. Chin recommended he add a vaporizer pen with a ratio of equal CBD to THC (1:1) rich in myrcene. After one inhalation, it gave him nausea relief within five minutes, and it also increased his appetite.

Cannabis worked well in Harold's case. He was able to eliminate three pharmaceutical medications. He no longer needed antinausea, anticonstipation, or pain medications. Harold preferred inhaling through a vaporizer ten minutes before meals for quick relief from nausea and a sublingual cannabis tincture midday to help with the cramping and bloating in his digestive tract. He also reported that, for the first time, he actually enjoyed eating and felt nourished and satiated by the food.

The following cannabinoids and terpenes may address nausea: THCA, THC, CBD, and myrcene.

CONDITION: PAIN AND SPASMS

Chef Andre, whose family owned a popular seafood restaurant, had a long history battling gout, a form of arthritis caused by a painful buildup of uric acid crystals in the joints. When he had his gout episodes, it would settle in his big toe, then his foot and ankle would swell up so much he would resort to submerging his foot in a bucket of ice just to relieve the pain and swelling. He had a hard time getting around and it affected his ability to work. When his attacks came on, they sent shooting pain up his leg as if he were stepping on blazing hot coals.

Chef Andre's sister, an oncology nurse, suggested he try a cannabis salve for the acute pain and swelling. He had to experiment with several brands of CBD-rich salves, and the salve he found most helpful was a full-spectrum extract of

250 milligram CBD enriched with emu oil. He applied this to his foot, and it helped with the localized redness, pain, and swelling. The salve also helped with the muscle cramping in his calf as the gout symptoms traveled up his leg.

Dr. Chin also recommended a CBD-rich, 20:1 ratio gel capsule (20 CBD to 1 THC), also rich in beta-carophyllene, to take orally to help reduce the pain so he could get back to work. He started with one gel capsule of 25 milligrams three times a day. He slowly increased his dose and found that he felt optimal relief when taking two capsules, three times a day, for a total of 150 milligrams per day.

Cannabinoids in cannabis prevent the release of inflammatory signals and work on the body's pain receptors, which is why cannabis products worked so well for Chef Andre's systemic pain and swelling. Cannabinoids in cannabis also target pain and inflammation in our bodies, similar to how NSAIDs such as ibuprofen do, without wreaking havoc on your gastrointestinal system.

The following cannabinoids and terpenes may reduce inflammation and lessen pain: THCA, THC, CBD, CBC, CBGA, CBG, pinene, beta-caryophyllene, geraniol, humulene, limonene, myrcene, terpineol, valencene.

CONDITION: ANXIETY AND PANIC ATTACKS

Alyssa had a five-year history of generalized anxiety disorder with panic attacks. She experienced waves of heart pounding, cold sweats, and tightness in her chest, and her hands shook uncontrollably. She was afraid of elevators and bridges as well as escalators and busy traffic intersections. She kept refilling the Xanax prescription her primary care doctor gave her, but realized she was trapped in a "revolving door" that she needed to stop.

Dr. Chin suggested she start taking a CBD-dominant sublingual tincture ratio of 20 CBD to 1 THC, rich in linalool. She started at 15 milligrams three times a day. She tried this for fourteen days and felt more relaxed and less anxious.

Dr. Chin advised her to add 1:6 THC sublingual tincture with a ratio of 1 CBD to 6 THC since THC and CBD in combination interact to enhance each other's effects. She started microdosing with the 1:6 tincture at night, beginning with a 1 milligram dose, right before bedtime. Dr. Chin discussed the side effects of too much THC, including increased heart rate, anxiety, euphoria, and drowsiness.

After trying this low-THC dose for three nights with no adverse effects, Alyssa experimented by adding the 1:6 THC tincture to her daytime 20:1 CBD dose. She used 1 milligram of 1:6 THC three times a day along with her usual 15 milligrams of CBD 20:1 three times a day. This cannabis regimen helped steady her nervous system and moderate her fears and anxiety.

Alyssa also wanted to stop the benzodiazepine medication upon which she was becoming increasingly dependent. Dr. Chin added a metered-dose inhaler of 1:6 THC infused with beta-carophyllene for emergent panic attacks. Each metered inhaled dose delivered 2 milligrams of THC. Alyssa was able to get out of situations where she felt crippled and unable to move. To modulate her body's reaction to stress, she found the prescribed cannabis regimen gave her sustained relief, reducing her fear and anxiety levels and lasting through the day without getting in the way of her work or social life.

Keeping up with the pace of our modern world can put our nervous systems into a constant heightened response. One of our own internal cannabis molecules, anandamide, helps us temper stress and balances our nervous system so we are not spiraling out of control on a high sympathetic nervous system overdrive.

The following cannabinoids and terpenes may address anxiety and panic attacks: THCV, CBD, beta-carophyllene, limonene, terpineol. THC may be used in smaller doses and in combination with CBD.

CONDITION: SEIZURES

"I feel like I am a victim in a Freddy Krueger movie," Jennifer said, referencing the infamous character from a 1980s horror movie who attacked victims in their dreams. Jennifer hated falling asleep. In fact, Jennifer hated sleeping. Ever since she was seven years old, right after she fell asleep, she would abruptly wake up with an epileptic seizure. She never had seizures during the daytime. The seizures would only occur soon after she fell into a sleep state. Jennifer's diagnosis was nocturnal seizures.

At thirty-seven years old, her nocturnal seizures were still not under control. She tried over a dozen antiseizure medications and even underwent two brain surgeries. Despite those treatments, she still had eighteen to twenty nighttime seizures per month.

After many months of trying different cannabis strains, Dr. Chin found a high-THC strain, 1 CBD to 20 THC, rich in beta-carophyllene that worked well for Jennifer, but then they faced an additional challenge of timing the intake of medication just right. On nights one to five, she started 1 milligram of 1:20 THC capsule before bedtime. This did not have an effect on decreasing her seizures.

> I feel like a new person. It was so exhausting. Every night, as I started to fall into a dream state, I was jolted awake, my arms and legs twitching and jerking, seeing flashes of light and then getting nauseous and dizzy. With the medical cannabis, I do not have to wake up with that fuzzy, hungover feeling. My muscles don't ache. I sleep, I feel free.

With Dr. Chin's guidance, she carefully increased to 1.5 milligrams for nights six through ten.

After careful titration and close monitoring of seizure activity by Dr. Chin and a neurologist, Jennifer titrated slowly to 2.5 milligrams of the 1:20 THC capsule about two and a half hours before bed. In addition to that dose, about thirty minutes before bed, she used a vaporizer form of 1:20 THC cannabis for fast-acting therapeutic effects of relaxation and drowsiness. By the time the cannabis metabolized in her body, it prevented the seizures that occurred at the onset of her sleep state.

After using cannabis for a year, Jennifer was having two to five seizures per month. If she stayed up late past her regular sleep schedule, or if she drank alcohol during dinner, she found it triggered her nocturnal seizures. Other than that, her nocturnal seizures were well controlled with cannabis medicine.

In one year, Jennifer lost about a hundred pounds, started exercising, and was able to get and keep a part-time job as an office assistant.

Cannabis has been used for centuries to treat seizures. On June 25, 2018, the USFDA approved the first prescription drug for seizures derived from cannabis, Epidiolex, specifically made from CBD extract. Dr. Orrin Devinsky, the principal investigator of the study behind Epidiolex, stated that "the CBD binds with a novel receptor in the brain and thereby dampens down too much electrical activity. CBD seems to be a relatively unique mechanism of action that's not shared by any of the existing seizure medications."

According to a study by the National Institute of Mental Health (NIMH), cannabis is also thought to have neuroprotective qualities. As a neuroprotectant, the CBD cannabinoid found in cannabis helps reduce damage to the brain and nervous system and encourages the growth and development of new neurons. This factor could explain why Jennifer found she was able to recover faster from the nighttime seizures and did not get a postseizure migraine.

The following cannabinoids and terpenes may address seizures (depending on the underlying cause): THC, THCA and THCV (for neuroprotective qualities), CBD, CBG, beta-carophyllene, geraniol, linalool.

Cannabis continues to be proven effective in treating acute conditions. Depending on the delivery method used, cannabis can be fast acting and long acting, especially when different methods are used together, such as vaping and taking cannabis in capsule form. Can cannabis also be effective for long-term, chronic conditions? Let's explore that next.

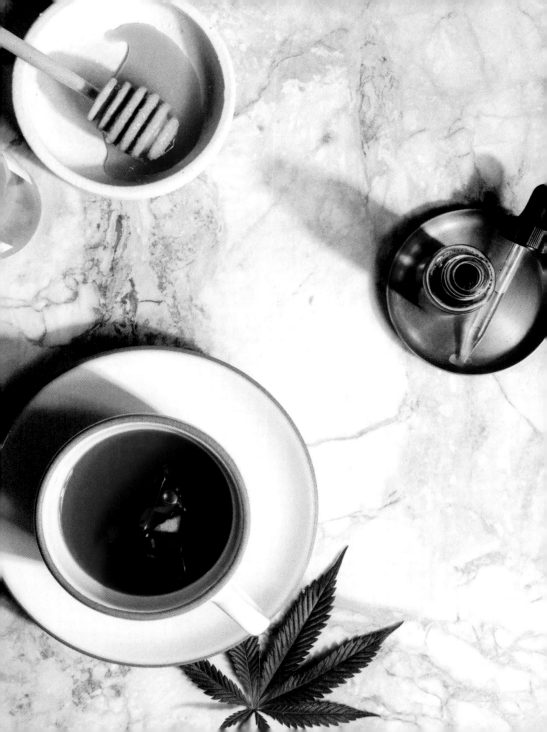

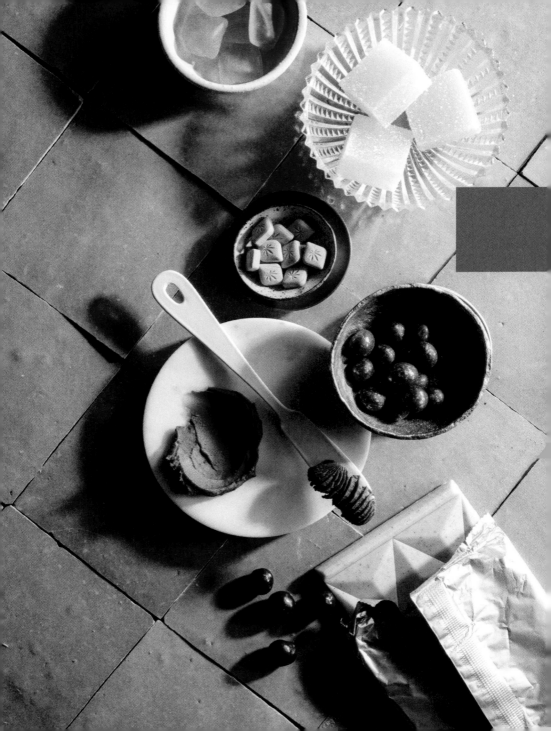

CHAPTER 10

Cannabis and Chronic Conditions

Many people experience acute health conditions in their lifetime and those experiences tend to get a lot of attention because they are often obvious and severe. Some people, however, are living with long-term, chronic conditions that can be just as debilitating. Some of these situations might seem minor or isolated but can chip away at their quality of life over time and affect many other aspects of their physical—and even mental—health. So where does cannabis fit in in terms of treating more chronic conditions? Here are some common chronic ailments and how some of Dr. Chin's patients are being treated for them.

CONDITION: INSOMNIA

According to the National Sleep Foundation, forty million Americans have a chronic sleep disorder. More than 60 percent of adults experience some type of sleep disturbance several nights a week. Cynthia started experiencing insomnia as she entered perimenopause at forty-six years old and began having difficulties falling asleep and staying asleep past 2 a.m.

At first, she tried over-the-counter medications, like Benadryl and Tylenol PM, but she frequently woke up in the morning with a headache and felt very dehydrated. Natural supplements such as melatonin, valerian root, and lavender oil didn't work for her nor did the sound machine she used to try to get her body and brain to wind down. Her primary care doctor prescribed a Z-drug sleep aid—a drug that is not a benzodiazepine but another class of medicine that acts in a similar way. Her doctor explained that insomnia was a normal part of life and that medication should "do the trick."

Within a week of taking it, she experienced parasomnias, a disruptive sleep disorder that could include talking or walking while still asleep, and that led to symptoms of anxiety throughout her day. Her doctor added a benzodiazepine, alprazolam, to help with the anxiety. Her doctor also recommended other types of insomnia medications, including various benzodiazepines and even antidepressants, but nothing resulted in a full, restorative night's sleep.

Cynthia went to Dr. Chin's office to ask for help. Dr. Chin recommended a vape pen to help her fall asleep quickly. Cynthia was uncomfortable using an inhaled form of cannabis.

As an alternative, Dr. Chin suggested a 1:6 THC sublingual linalool and myrcene spray formula that delivered 1 milligram per dose of cannabis for fast onset of action to help her wind down and get to sleep quicker. She also recommended an additional 1:3 THC cannabis gel capsule of 1 milligram to help her sleep through the night so she would not have to worry about getting up at 2 or 3 a.m.

After the first night of taking cannabis, Cynthia woke up feeling very groggy in the morning and tossed and turned all night. She was having vivid dreams and did not feel well rested at all. In fact, she reported feeling more tired and anxious. Dr. Chin concluded that the extra cannabis gel capsule was too much, and she was experiencing the side effects of the THC. When Cynthia stopped the 1:3 capsule and only took the 1:6 sublingual spray, she slept like a baby.

> "For the first time in over eighteen months, I had seven hours of uninterrupted sleep, and woke up feeling refreshed. I also began to notice my daytime anxiety levels were manageable, and I was more resilient in coping with stress. I feel like someone pressed the 'reset button' in my life."

Why does cannabis work for insomnia during perimenopause? High estrogen levels during perimenopause can produce heightened levels of anxiety in women and an interruption in their sleep cycle. High levels of estrogen also inhibit GABA, a naturally occurring brain chemical that directs neurons to slow down or stop firing. GABA is a calming neurotransmitter that helps to induce sleep, relax muscles, and reduce anxiety. In essence, GABA directs the body to power down.

Cannabis modulates the neurotransmitter GABA, helping return it to its more normal functions. Careful cannabis dosing helped free Cynthia from the racing thoughts that caused disrupted sleep and panicked awakenings at all hours of the night. She no longer needed additional medications to wake up feeling rested or to get through her day.

The following cannabinoids and terpenes may address insomnia: THC, CBD (particularly paired with THC), CBN, linalool, myrcene.

CONDITION: NERVE PAIN

Danny has had type 2 diabetes for over ten years. He has kept his chronic condition under control following a balanced whole foods diet and limiting his intake of processed foods. For the last year, he found it difficult to walk and stay active due to nerve pain in both his legs. He described the sensation in his legs and feet as a burning, fiery pain. His condition was affecting his ability to move around and hampering his ability to travel.

Danny tried various medications to address his nerve pain, including gabapentin, pregabalin, and amitriptyline. Each of these medications worked for a short while. The main side effect, however, was that they made Danny extremely sleepy and higher doses gave him negative cognitive effects. He also tried myriad alternative therapies, like massage, acupuncture, foot soaks, TENS unit stimulation, and custom-made foot orthotics.

Dr. Chin suggested a 1:1 CBD to THC oral tablet with pinene and a transdermal patch to address the burning nerve pain. With the entourage effect, CBD counterbalances the euphoric side effects of THC. The 1:1 ratio is commonly used in elderly patients with nerve pain. THC is especially helpful with acute, burning nerve pain and CBD helps with the underlying inflammatory aspect of the neuropathy.

Danny started low and slow. He began with taking the 1:1 CBD to THC tablet at night before bed, just in case it caused drowsiness or euphoria. When he realized he was able to tolerate it well, he found that taking one capsule four times a day was optimal for his pain. Within a couple of weeks, Danny found that his nerve pain was reduced.

He continued to use the gabapentin at night but only needed a fraction of the dose. He used the cannabis tablet and transdermal patch during the daytime and did not feel sedated, nor did the cannabis treatment cause brain fog.

The majority of existing data about cannabis for treating discomfort actually comes from patients with chronic neuropathic pain arising from a variety of conditions. In a review of thirty-eight randomized-controlled clinical review trials, more than 70 percent of these studies concluded that cannabinoids in cannabis had statistically significant pain-relieving effects compared to placebo. Cannabis is an effective treatment of nerve pain with both anti-inflammatory effects and unique pain-relieving attributes.

The following cannabinoids and terpenes may address nerve pain (as well as have anti-inflammatory and analgesic effects): THC, THCA, CBD, CBC, beta-caryophyllene, geraniol, humulene, limonene, myrcene, terpineol, valencene.

CONDITION: AUTOIMMUNE DISORDERS

Insomnia, inflammation, and pain reduction aren't the only chronic health conditions that cannabis can address. Cannabinoids in cannabis can bind to our CB2 receptors, the receptors found in our immune systems, and produce positive effects. The immune system is made up of a network of cells, tissues, and organs that work together to protect the body against viruses, bacteria, and other foreign organisms. Sometimes, our immune systems can backfire on us, resulting in an autoimmune disease where the immune system attacks the healthy cells in our bodies by mistake.

Lupus is a chronic autoimmune disease that can damage any part of the body, including our skin, joints, and organs. The Lupus Foundation of America estimates that 1.5 million Americans, and at least five million people around the world, have a form of lupus. Sophia was diagnosed with lupus right after college. She spent most of her college years feeling tired, fighting the flu, and having recurrent bouts of shingles. When she graduated, her symptoms of hair loss, headaches, fatigue, and skin rashes only escalated. After speaking with her aunt who suffered from similar symptoms and had been recently diagnosed with an autoimmune disease, Sophia decided to see a rheumatologist.

Sophia's symptoms were constantly fluctuating. One day, she would have a rash all over her body, the next day she couldn't get out of bed because her knees were swollen. Sophia's doctor prescribed steroids and immunosuppressive medication. That worked well for over seven years. She stopped having flare-ups, and her symptoms were no longer a problem. Sophia finished medical school, passing her exams with flying colors, and became a physician. Her disease was under control until the birth of her first child.

Pregnancy and childbirth caused a massive flare-up of her lupus and sent her into a whirlwind of taking multiple medications to try to control her symptoms. Her previous medication regimen did not work at all. In fact, after trying multiple immunosuppressant medications, nothing seemed to help anymore. The only thing that provided her with any relief was a high-dose steroid. Sophia and her doctor understood the negative long-term consequences of steroid use, including osteoporosis, diabetes, and increasing her risk of infections. At a medical conference, Sophia heard about cannabinoids and their immunosuppressive properties. She wondered if cannabis could help wean her off steroids.

Dr. Chin started Sophia on a cannabis tincture that was higher in CBD than THC, a 20 CBD to 1 THC ratio with limonene. She started with 15 milligrams of tincture once a day. Every seven days, she carefully titrated her dose by increasing it by 5 milligrams until she felt her lupus symptoms improve. After a month, she found her optimal therapeutic dosage to be 35 milligrams of tincture every six hours.

> "The joints in my hands and feet are not swollen anymore. I can actually make a fist! I have less fatigue, joint and muscle pain, morning stiffness."

Dr. Chin also put Sophia on an autoimmune protocol (AIP) diet, eliminating foods that can cause inflammation, such as grains, legumes, dairy, refined sugar, and processed foods. Instead, Sophia consumed meats, vegetables except for those in the nightshade family (tomatoes, potatoes), and fermented foods, similar to a paleo diet but more limited. After three months of using the CBD tincture and changing her eating habits, Sophia and Dr. Chin worked with Sophia's rheumatologist to carefully wean her off the steroid medication.

Cannabinoids can be promising immunosuppressive agents in the therapy of autoimmune disorders. Cannabinoids help calm down an overactive immune system by working directly on cells and biological processes that regulate the immune system. Cannabis seems to decrease inflammation in the body by suppressing certain parts of the immune system.

The following cannabinoids and terpenes may address symptoms from autoimmune disorders as well as have anti-inflammatory effects (depending on the underlying cause): THCA, CBD with smaller amounts of THC, CBC, beta-caryophyllene, geraniol, humulene, limonene, myrcene, terpineol, valencene.

CONDITION: CANCER

James was fifty-eight years old and being treated for pancreatic cancer at a top cancer hospital in New York City. He did well with the initial surgery and chemotherapy and was using the opiate pain medication and antinausea medication his oncologist prescribed. When he got through his fourth round of chemo, things began to shift for him. He started losing his appetite and his pain level increased dramatically. James was also having trouble sleeping through the night, as a side effect of the chemo included insomnia.

Because James could not tolerate the taste of tinctures and his digestive tract did not metabolize cannabis pills well, Dr. Chin started him on a 1:6 THC vape pen with myrcene to quell his nausea and pain and to help decrease his anxiety. James used two different vape pens with various cannabinoid profiles. He used 1:6 THC vape pen for the daytime and 1:20 THC vaporizer pen with myrcene and beta-carophyllene before bedtime. The 1:6 THC vape formulations helped to decrease pain during

> My appetite began to come back. The cannabis gave me the munchies. I started to crave food and put on weight. It also helped me manage my insomnia. After chemo, I would feel both exhausted and wide awake at the same time. The cannabis helped me relax, sleep, and eat.

the day without making him too drowsy or euphoric, and the 1:20 THC vape pen for bedtime helped him with sleep and nausea.

Due to the quick onset of action—between five and ten minutes—James was able to get immediate feedback on how his body responded and how much cannabis dosage he needed daily. Two to three days postchemo, he found he needed to use the vape pen more often.

Cannabis is the only antinausea medicine that also increases appetite, aids with sleep, and elevates mood, something that is not easy to do when someone is facing a chronic and life-threatening illness. While doctors often write five different prescription medications—painkiller, antinausea, antianxiety, appetite stimulant, and a sedative—that may or may not interact with one another, they could recommend trying one plant medicine first, cannabis, and address all five symptoms at once.

The following cannabinoids and terpenes may address symptoms from chemo, including nausea and insomnia: THCA, THC, CBD, beta-caryophyllene, linalool, myrcene.

Cannabis is not a cure-all or silver bullet for everything that ails you, but more and more research shows that it is effective in addressing chronic health conditions by relieving symptoms and also addressing and modulating your body's internal systems. By getting to the root of many disorders—an out-of-balance, poorly nourished endocannabinoid system—cannabis can offer deeper, more lasting relief.

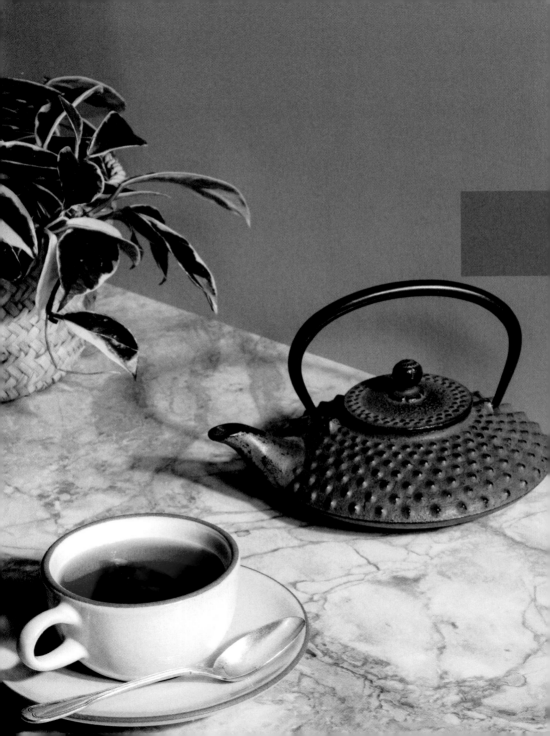

CHAPTER 11

Cannabis and Your Mind

We've explained how acute and chronic health conditions can be addressed with cannabis, but what about mental conditions? How does cannabis affect the mind? According to psychopharmacologist and psychiatrist Dr. Julie Holland, who is also author of the book *The Truth About the Drugs You're Taking, the Sleep You're Missing, the Sex You're Not Having, and What's Really Making You Crazy*, your body's natural "cannabis molecules" make you resistant to stress, similar to the way your endorphin system provides natural pain relief.

Stress can have a devastating impact on our bodies, including an increased risk for diabetes, heart disease, high blood pressure, and a compromised immune system. Stress can also impact our mental health. Stress, and chemical imbalances in our brains, can lead to anxiety and depression, among other mental disorders.

Preclinical studies show that our endocannabinoid system (ECS) helps modulate endocrine and neuronal responses to stress; that is, it affects how our hormone-producing glands and our brain's neurons deal with the chemicals released—adrenaline and cortisol—when we're stressed. When our bodies face stressful situations, our ECS also kicks into gear to help us balance our nervous system. Scientists in Wisconsin, Illinois, and Germany found that people with higher anandamide levels in their system could tolerate life stressors better.

As we explained previously, anandamide was the first endocannabinoid found in mammals, referred to as the "bliss molecule" (see page 33), and as part of our ECS, it affects pain, appetite, memory, fertility, and depression. Cannabis, particularly the cannabinoid CBD, can increase anandamide in our system. In the simplest terms, more anandamide means less stress, more bliss. In practice, cannabis can address more complex mental conditions. Let's look specifically at post-traumatic stress disorder (PTSD), depression, and ADHD through the experiences of some of Dr. Chin's patients.

CONDITION: POST-TRAUMATIC STRESS DISORDER

Michael is a retired NYPD officer and was a first responder after the 9/11 attack on New York City. Nearly two decades later, he was unable to shake the memories of that terrifying day and its aftermath. Michael had the most trouble at bedtime. When he closed his eyes at night to go to sleep, he replayed the disaster in his mind over and over again. If he was lucky and his sleep medication worked, he could drift to sleep. A few hours later, nightmares forced him awake. He darted out of bed in a cold sweat, out of breath, clenching his chest. During the day, he had trouble concentrating.

Michael was diagnosed with PTSD and began seeing a therapist every week. His psychiatrist prescribed two antidepressants, a benzodiazepine, and a sleep aid. After many years of trial and error, the combination of these medications helped him with his daily jitteriness and debilitating panic attacks, but he still felt helpless, alone, and empty. He also had a history of suicidal thoughts.

Michael's older brother, a war veteran, suggested Michael try cannabis to help ease his anxiety and help him forget the painful memories. As part of the NYPD, Michael spent years making marijuana arrests. When he came into Dr. Chin's office, he said, "I can't understand why taking an illicit and highly addictive drug would help me move on and lead a productive life." He believed marijuana was a threat to society and ruined families. He was only open to learning more about cannabis because he saw how much it helped his older brother lead a normal life. He said he was willing to try it for exactly thirty days, but he stipulated, "I don't want to smoke it, I don't want to get high, and I don't want to sit on the couch with the munchies."

Dr. Chin suggested a bedtime formula of 1:6 THC sublingual spray with linalool at 1 milligram for the first week to help Michael get a full night's sleep without the interruption of nightmares. At the second week, Dr. Chin added a daytime 20:1 CBD sublingual tincture with limonene at 25 milligrams two times a day to help Michael clear the negative memories. Dr. Chin worked closely with Michael's psychiatrist and psychotherapist to monitor his progress. Michael kept a detailed journal as well (for more on keeping your own journal, see page 100).

Michael found the 1:6 THC kept him up at night and increased his nightmares. He stopped the nighttime THC and continued with the 20:1 CBD during the day. After a few weeks of CBD use, Michael found it really upset his stomach and created symptoms of diarrhea. When he stopped the CBD, his stomach upset disappeared. Dr. Chin recommended another brand of 10:1 CBD with pinene at the same dose of 25 milligrams two times a day. Michael found relief with this new formula and CBD brand.

After the first month, Michael's therapist reported that she felt he was more relaxed, grounded, and present, and their sessions were more supportive for him. Michael also noticed a difference.

After about six months of medical cannabis use, Michael's psychiatrist was able to reduce his medication to one antidepressant medication and the occasional benzodiazepine. He was able to stop taking his sleep aid completely.

According to two different studies from NYU and Vanderbilt University, PTSD patients have been shown to have lower levels of the "bliss molecule," anandamide, compared to people without PTSD. Anandamide in our ECS helps clear painful memories and reduce our stress levels. A side effect of cannabis can be short-term memory loss, and this side effect of

> "I started to feel more like myself again. I get a better quality of sleep with fewer nightmares, which really helps me be more productive during the day. Overall, I feel a better sense of well-being, less nervous and on edge."

forgetting benefits patients such as Michael. With cannabis use, the haunting and exhausting memories stopped replaying in his mind, finally giving him some peace.

The following cannabinoids and terpenes may address symptoms from PTSD: THCA, THC, CBD, limonene, linalool.

CONDITION: DEPRESSION

Depression is a complex neuropsychiatric disease that involves many factors, including genetic predisposition, stress, trauma, and medical illness and medication. Major Depressive Disorder (MDD) is the most prevalent psychiatric disorder in the world. MDD is also known as clinical depression, unipolar depression, or, simply, depression. The World Health Organization predicts that, by the year 2030, depression will be the leading cause of disability worldwide.

Due to the fact that depression is such a multifaceted and dynamic disease process, combining several treatment modalities is often necessary to get to the root cause of it. Cannabis can be one of those methods of treatment, and one of Dr. Chin's patients discovered how effective—but also complex—treating depression with cannabis can be.

For as long as Angela could remember, she always felt sad. When other kids were giggling and running around in the playground, she felt a "heaviness" inside and an overwhelming sense of doom and sadness. She was a quiet child and often sat alone. Depression ran in her family. Her mother, grandmother, aunts, and cousins had a history of depression. Angela began taking medication for depression at the age of eight.

As an adult, Angela cycled through more than a dozen anti-depressant medications and all the alternative therapies she could find. She even visited a shaman in the mountains of Peru in hopes of pulling herself out of the dark abyss of sadness. While vacationing with her cousins, they offered her a pot brownie. Angela was extremely hesitant about trying it, recalling a frightening, uncomfortable experience she had as a teen with cannabis. She took a morsel of the brownie, the size of her thumbnail. To her surprise, the effect was positive.

Angela was so excited she took three brownie pieces with her and tried consuming some again the next evening. This time, she did not feel the same effect, so she took a second piece within the same hour. Ten minutes later, she broke out in a cold sweat and felt nauseous. Angela brought the rest of the brownie pieces into Dr. Chin's office and described the relief she had with the first bite and said she wanted to find an equivalent cannabis formula.

Edibles or baked cannabis products are less likely to produce consistent, standardized dosing. Dr. Chin suggested, as an alternative, quick-dissolving 20:1 CBD cannabis tablets to start. After about a week of taking 25 milligrams three times a day, Angela did not find relief. Dr. Chin suggested she try adding THC-rich formula 1:6 with linalool in the form of a sublingual tincture. One spray delivered 1 milligram of THC.

Angela tried the first dose before bed in case it made her drowsy or euphoric. She did find it sedating, so she used only the THC formula at bedtime. She began titrating carefully by increments of 1 milligram each night until she felt symptom relief. She continued the CBD during the day. Dr. Chin explained that even though she didn't feel any immediate relief from the CBD after a week, continuing to take the CBD formula would help her balance her endocannabinoid system (ECS).

Dr. Chin and Angela worked together to come up with a safe microdosing plan so Angela would consume smaller doses of cannabis over the course of the day to get the benefits of the plant's compounds without potentially unpleasant side effects. After about twelve weeks of careful journaling and experimenting, Angela found her optimal therapeutic dosage of 3 milligrams of 1:6 THC at bedtime and 75 milligrams of CBD, three times per day.

Antidepressant medications used to treat patients with depression work by boosting and modulating the concentration of neurotransmitters. Neurotransmitters are chemical messengers in the nervous system that help send messages from one cell to another. Researchers have pinpointed the following neurotransmitters as key players in depression: acetylcholine, serotonin, norepinephrine, dopamine, glutamate, and GABA.

While there are limited studies on how the ECS affects depression, researchers are recognizing that the way cannabis affects our ECS does contribute to the complex neuronal network in our brains and can be applied in the treatment of depression.

Researchers at McGill University found that low doses of THC increase serotonin, but high doses of THC can cause a decrease in serotonin that could worsen depression. Angela worked with Dr. Chin to find her optimal therapeutic dosage of cannabis that happened to be a microdose. Everyone is different in terms of how their bodies and brains process cannabis and how it may or may not address symptoms of depression. Angela's psychiatrist continues to manage the conventional medication that Angela takes along with cannabis.

The following cannabinoids and terpenes may address symptoms of depression: THC, CBD, limonene, linalool.

CONDITION: ATTENTION DEFICIT/HYPERACTIVITY DISORDER

Any neurological disorder can be stressful and debilitating, whether it is PTSD or depression or even attention deficit/hyperactivity disorder (ADHD). Although the research for ADHD and cannabis is still in its infancy, a study of thirty patients in Germany suggests that, for adult patients with ADHD who experience side effects or do not benefit from standard medication, cannabis may be an effective and well-tolerated alternative. Dr. Chin's patient, Sue, was about to discover this for herself.

> "CBD helps me stay on track; I feel focused, less distracted and ultimately that makes me less anxious."

Sue wasn't diagnosed with ADHD until she was an adult. Sue's psychiatrist described her ADHD brain as a Ferrari engine, moving at lightning speed but, unfortunately, she had bicycle pedals for brakes. Sue took her ADHD prescription medication religiously, and it helped her focus without getting consumed by fatigue by midday. Sue was also a medical cannabis patient.

After experimenting with various cannabinoid formulas and ratios, from CBD-rich 20:1, 1:1 (CBD to THC), 1:3 THC, 1:6 THC, and finally 1:20 THC, she found that the higher the THC, the more anxious she felt. CBD-rich formulas such as 20:1 work best for her but only in small amounts. Her optimal dosage is 5 milligrams CBD once per day.

Sue uses a 20:1 CBD metered inhaler that delivers the 5 milligrams each time. This small dose is helpful in keeping her concentration sharp and her energy levels up. She finds anything more than 5 milligrams sedating.

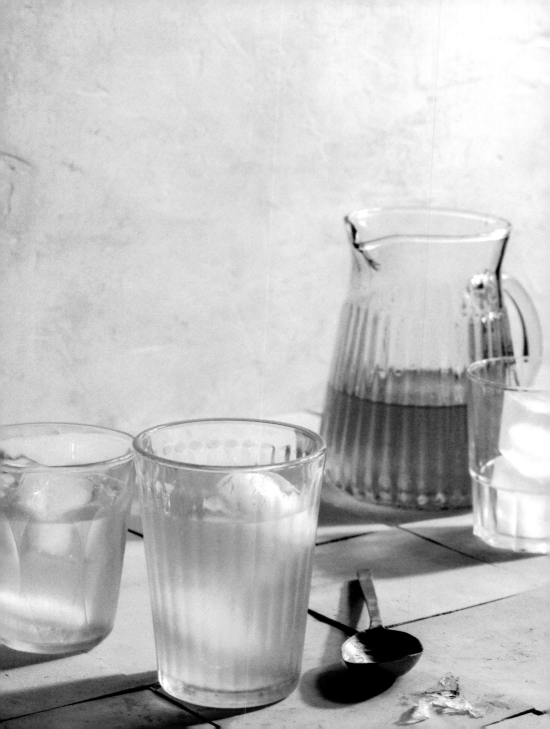

According to the National Institutes of Health, ADHD may be genetic. Sue wondered if cannabis could help her nine-year-old son Jared with his ADHD and behaviorial issues like it helped her. While a healthier endocannabinoid system can improve the quality of life for patients, treating certain pediatric illnesses with cannabis must be handled with caution because there are little to no long-term clinical studies on the therapeutic uses of cannabis with children. The American Academy of Pediatrics recommends behavior therapy as the first line treatment for young ADHD patients.

Cannabis can have a significant effect on the young, developing brain. A healthy, normal functioning child or teenager should not use cannabis. When a young person uses cannabis, administering exogenous—or "from outside of the body"—phytocannabinoids can overwhelm their highly sensitive endocannabinoid system.

While our ECS is indeed responsible for balancing and providing homeostasis within our bodies, preclinical studies show that phytocannabinoids can cause our own ECS receptors to downregulate, or reduce. This effect can throw off the very system that regulates our brains as well as our immune and endocrine systems. Translation: Cannabis intake can result in impaired attention, memory learning, and decision making in an underdeveloped brain.

In 2017, a small, randomized controlled trial followed patients with ADHD taking a cannabinoid medication. The study did show improvements in their ADHD symptoms and the results also suggest that adults who take cannabinoids for ADHD experience the side effects less than children. This may help to explain why patients such as Sue find that as an adult, medical cannabis does not give her unwanted cognitive side effects. Instead, cannabis helps give her energy and focus, and helps her to be more productive.

The following cannabinoids and terpenes may address symptoms of ADHD: THC, CBD, linalool, myrcene.

As you can see from these patient stories, cannabis dosages and formulas vary from individual to individual. There is no one size fits all. Finding your optimal therapeutic dosage takes time and patience. All patients are encouraged to follow the dosing guidelines on page 98 and journal results. If you don't feel significant improvements within four weeks, make adjustments in formula, delivery method, or ratio of cannabinoids as well as terpene content.

We've now talked about how cannabis can be effective for addressing mental health conditions and disorders, from ADHD to post-traumatic stress disorder and depression. Cannabinoids and terpenes contained within cannabis can nourish and modulate the endocannabinoid system in a multitude of ways that can be helpful for acute, chronic, or severe physical and mental health issues. In the next chapter, we'll look at a number of ways cannabis and CBD can play a positive role in our overall health and wellness.

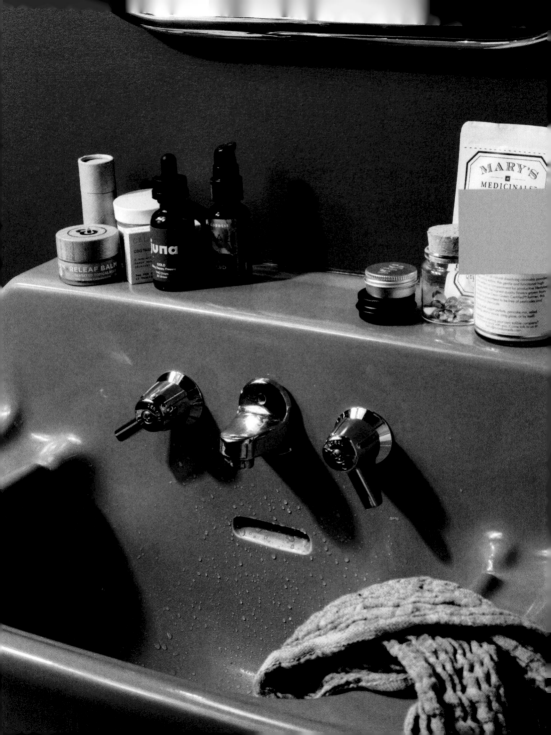

CHAPTER 12

Cannabis and Well-Being

As we've explained, cannabis and CBD can be effective in addressing myriad physical and mental health issues, both chronic and acute. Cannabis and CBD can also be used to optimize your overall feeling of well-being. The cannabis plant can provide your body and brain with beneficial cannabinoids and terpenes, each of which can have a positive impact on your health. Nourishing your endocannabinoid system can be the missing link in your overall quest for living a better, healthier life or simply feeling good.

Being in good health makes everything you encounter in life seem more manageable. With more rest, less pain, less stress, and more joy, you are able to better handle whatever comes your way. Following are a number of areas of general wellness where cannabis and CBD can play a positive role.

SELF-CARE

In 2015, the American Psychological Association put out a report stating that surveyed adults reported that stress had a negative impact on their mental and physical health, and many did not feel they were doing enough to manage their stress. While money and work were cited as the top two stressors in their lives, half of the respondents brought up two new stressors: personal health concerns and health problems affecting their family. If cannabis can be effective in improving health, it stands to reason that some common stressors may be reduced.

If you've looked closely at self-care as a route to better health and well-being, you may have heard that the three critical pillars of self-care are sleep, fitness, and nutrition. Getting a good night's sleep, adding more movement into your day, and eating right can fortify your body and brain to handle life's stressors. Sleep is critical. Without it, all other aspects of your life can be affected. If cannabis can help you get a better night's sleep, that alone could greatly improve your ability to cope with stressors and find the motivation to get more exercise and improve your eating habits.

Cannabis and CBD can be part of a regular self-care routine, with or without THC. Consuming cannabis therapeutically, but also recreationally, can enhance wellness, with the major difference being the end goal: health benefits versus getting high. Based on the studies we've read, cannabis is a healthier way to relax than with alcohol or drugs, like sedatives or opioids, and with far fewer side effects.

You don't have to consume cannabis for self-care, although a nice cup of THC and CBD tea might be quite calming. You can integrate cannabis and CBD into general personal care with activities such as these:

- ▶ Treat your skin with a cannabis or CBD-infused topical such as a lotion, cream, lip balm, face serum, or face mask (this is also good for preventing and managing acne).
- ▶ Soak your body or your feet in a cannabis or CBD bath using an infused bath bomb or oil containing a sedating cannabinoid (like CBN) or terpene (like linalool).
- ▶ Wash your body and hair with cannabis- or CBD-infused soaps, shampoos, and conditioners.
- ▶ Create a relaxing atmosphere with cannabis- and terpene-scented candles and room sprays.
- ▶ Ask your partner to give you a massage using THC-infused or CBD-containing massage oil.

Or, of course, you can opt to consume cannabis in your favorite form at the end of the day to relax and unwind.

Keep in mind that just because a beauty or home product contains CBD it does not mean it will have a major impact on your health. Companies that add CBD to products with otherwise harmful ingredients won't suddenly become healthier with CBD. Use the same criteria for purchasing cannabis and CBD products as you would other products that you apply or use. If you like organic products, seek out organic cannabis or CBD products. If you can't find products that state the cannabis or CBD was grown organically, look at the other ingredients to see if they are organic. Watch out for ingredients that you can't pronounce or that are known or suspected to be carcinogenic, such as propylene glycol, just as you would when reading a processed food label.

Unless you buy beauty or home products at a licensed cannabis dispensary or store, they will not legally contain THC. Unless you consume a product containing THC in a manner that gets it into your bloodstream (see pages 89 to 90), adding cannabis to home products such as candles or room sprays won't get you high.

As with any product you use on your body or in your home, test a small amount at first to make sure you—or anyone in your home—does not have an allergic reaction. We'll cover more about bringing cannabis-based products into your home in the next chapter.

PHYSICAL FITNESS

Managing stress can do wonders for your health. Staying active is also part of maintaining overall wellness. Cannabis and CBD can be useful tools for athletes but also anyone who is exercising, playing sports, training for a sporting event, or otherwise physically exerting themselves. Think of the various therapeutic effects of cannabis and CBD that we've discussed in this book and how they might help while you work out:

▶ Anti-inflammatory—reduces inflammation from joint, muscle, and tendon overuse or injury

▶ Antispasmodic—reduces muscle spasms

▶ Pain reducer—eases soreness and pain

By reducing inflammation and pain, cannabis and CBD can aid in recovery postworkout and continued healing.

An appropriate dose of THC can help you "get into the zone" and focus or even relax into your workout. Some physical activities that can be enhanced with cannabis include workouts on the elliptical, treadmill, stationary bike or other repetitive exercise, yoga, walking, hiking, jogging, and mountain biking away from traffic and on well-groomed trails. Activities that require complex coordination are probably not the best ones to do while consuming cannabis, but you should be fine taking nonpsychotropic CBD.

When it comes to THC and exercise, make sure you know your dose and already have a preferred delivery method so you are aware of how you tend to feel after you consume and how long effects set in for you. Exercising while high can be relaxing; however, you don't want to be so high that you lose your balance or control of your motor skills, resulting in injury. Focus more on microdosing than consuming a larger amount that can produce a stronger high that might cause you to lose some depth perception or balance, resulting in a fall.

A safe option for a workout after consuming cannabis is a walk or jog around your neighborhood or a workout at home. Unless you are at a workout facility that legally allows consumption, do not consume in a public place. Instead, opt for a slower-acting cannabis product with THC, such as an edible or ingestible (like a tablet or capsule), and head straight to the gym or yoga studio so you are not driving when the THC takes effect. Plan to avoid driving for several hours after you've consumed to ensure you aren't driving intoxicated.

Taking CBD before or after your workout is discreet and not mind-altering. The inflammation and pain reduction properties of CBD can be useful in supporting recovery after a workout. Instead of popping a few ibuprofen that can irritate your stomach and strain your liver, a supportive dose of CBD can take the edge off of aches from muscle strain and promote healing. After you've gone through a thoughtful product selection process using the tips and guidelines in chapters 6 and 7, you should know what strains or products, cannabinoids and terpenes, and ratios and doses work best for you. Keep in mind that what might be effective before bedtime for sleep will be different from what helps you with a workout and recovery. Calibrate your dose through trial and error over time but start lower than you might typically take, then increase the amount incrementally.

THCV as an Appetite Suppressant

When you think of using cannabis or getting high, you might immediately think about getting the munchies, those uncontrollable cravings for food, particularly sweet or salty items. Big bag of potato chips, anyone? The munchies are THC at work. Cannabis can be very useful for treating nausea and increasing appetite, particularly in people with wasting diseases or going through chemotherapy and suffering from side effects that make eating difficult. Another of the cannabinoids in cannabis, however, can act as an appetite suppressant. Tetrahydrocannabivarin, or THCV, is not formed from CBGA like THCA. THCV is psychotropic in high doses but not in low doses. In addition to appetite suppression, THCV also reduces insulin resistance and regulates blood sugar levels.

As with any cannabis product, ask a budtender at your trusted dispensary, check manufacturer websites, and read reviews and ratings online from trusted sources to find products that are being made with particular cannabinoids or terpenes. Some strains, concentrates, tinctures, tablets, and oral absorption products are manufactured to specifically contain THCV. Some strains that may contain high levels of THCV include Tangie, Durban Poison, and Girl Scout Cookies.

IN THE BEDROOM

Another physical activity where cannabis and CBD can be useful is sex. Cannabis has been used for centuries in some cultures as an aphrodisiac. In Ayurvedic practices dating back to 2000 BCE, cannabis in small quantities was used as both pain reliever and aphrodisiac. Ancient Tantric sexual practices included the consumption of *bhang*, a mixture of cannabis leaves, flowers, and stems blended with milk, water, and spices such as cardamom.

Sex involves a complex set of physical, mental, and emotional reactions that can be affected by cannabis or CBD. Cannabis can promote the following, all of which could enhance your sex life:

▶ Increased relaxation

▶ Reduced anxiety

▶ Lowered inhibitions

▶ Increased hormone production

▶ Increased sexual arousal

▶ Increased sensitivity in your erogenous zones

▶ Enhanced creativity

People may experience sexual health issues at different stages of their lives. A common sexual issue for people, either those going through perimenopause or menopause or those who have entered menopause prematurely from illness or hysterectomy, is vaginal pain during sex. Cannabis can quickly reduce the sensation of pain when smoked, vaped, or ingested, but even more effective is a topical vaginal cream, spray, lubricant, or suppository containing a concentration of THC, like the products from Foria. Cannabis topicals or suppositories manufactured for vaginal use and applied to the vagina and in and around the vaginal canal can offer near-immediate pain relief, increase blood flow to the area, and enhance sexual pleasure. None of the topical or vaginal forms of delivery of THC should affect your brain or make you high, although the lower region of your body may feel very relaxed.

Another common sexual issue faced by some people is erectile dysfunction. Whether stemming from a physical, mental, or emotional cause, erectile dysfunction can put a damper on a sexual experience that can carry over to future encounters. Cannabis can reduce performance anxiety and enhance sexual pleasure. The penis has cannabinoid receptors, so it can be affected by cannabis consumption or application.

Too much of a good thing is usually not a good thing, and in the case of THC, getting too high can dampen sensitivity, interfere with erections, and increase the chance of mental distraction and sleepiness. Unfortunately, there is not yet sufficient research to clearly demonstrate how cannabis consumption affects us during sex. Reports have found that regular consumers of cannabis have 20 percent more sex than nonconsumers. One report concluded that cannabis did not impair sexual function.

If vaping or smoking before sex, pick strains in flower or concentrate form depending on the effects you are seeking to enhance your sex life. If you're looking for energy, euphoria, and stimulation, sativas are the way to go, and you may get more of a head high from strains such as Ultimate Trainwreck and Green Crack or a sativa/indica hybrid, like Sour Dream or Sour Diesel. Keep in mind that a sativa can also keep you awake, even after a night of great sex. Indicas such as Granddaddy Purple or Blue Cheese can increase arousal and the duration or intensity of orgasms but too much can be sleep inducing.

If you're using a manufactured product for sexual enhancement, such as In the Moment oral spray by Karezza, follow the instructions, including how soon before sex to take it, usually at least twenty minutes for topicals, less time for tinctures and sublinguals, and even less for smoking or vaping.

If your partner isn't interested in trying cannabis-enhanced sex, you can still partake to enhance your own performance and pleasure, although open communication is recommended. In the same way you discuss condoms or the use of lubricants or sex toys, talking about cannabis for sex should be done openly and honestly.

Taking cannabis internally through edibles, ingestibles, or oral absorption can be discreet and not offensive to a partner who isn't personally a fan of cannabis. You definitely do not have to smoke or vape cannabis to enhance sex, but if you do, watch out for any flammable material in the bedroom. While going for hot sex, make sure you don't start a fire!

PRODUCTIVITY, CREATIVITY, AND JOY

With the wider availability of a variety of cannabis strains and products, producing different effects is more possible than ever. While we've talked extensively about addressing chronic or acute health conditions, we haven't yet touched on recreational use or consuming cannabis for the sheer pleasure. Some people simply enjoy how cannabis makes them feel without thinking about the added health benefits.

Laughter is proven to be good medicine, and consuming cannabis to laugh or feel blissful can improve one's sense of overall well-being. Look for a hybrid strain that can provide a nice balance of euphoria and relaxation, such as Girl Scout Cookies (indica dominant) or Jack Herer (sativa dominant).

Some people also find that sativa strains that are mentally stimulating—like Cinex, Sour Diesel, and Green Crack—help them focus and be more productive. On the flip side, some people prefer a more relaxed focus, a zoning-in feeling, from strains such as Blueberry Headband or Goo. A relaxed high might also help unleash creativity that can often be hampered by self-critique and performance anxiety.

AGING WELL

As we age, we experience myriad changes in our bodies and brains. Our bodily functions can become impaired, our hormone production becomes irregular, and the daily stressors of life can lead to disease. Given the already documented therapeutic benefits of cannabis and CBD, it's no wonder that boomers and seniors are increasingly trying and using cannabis.

One study saw an increase in cannabis use among people living with two or more chronic conditions, and an even greater increase in people living with depression, all of which could, in some cases, be attributed to aging. With cannabis becoming legal and available in more places, it stands to reason that older people may seek out the therapeutic benefits of cannabis and CBD to reduce their use of prescription medications that may have unwanted side effects.

Another study took a look at the patterns of cannabis consumption among Americans aged fifty and older and reported a more than 70 percent increase between 2006 and 2013. Ninety-one percent of the seniors surveyed said they would recommend cannabis to others.

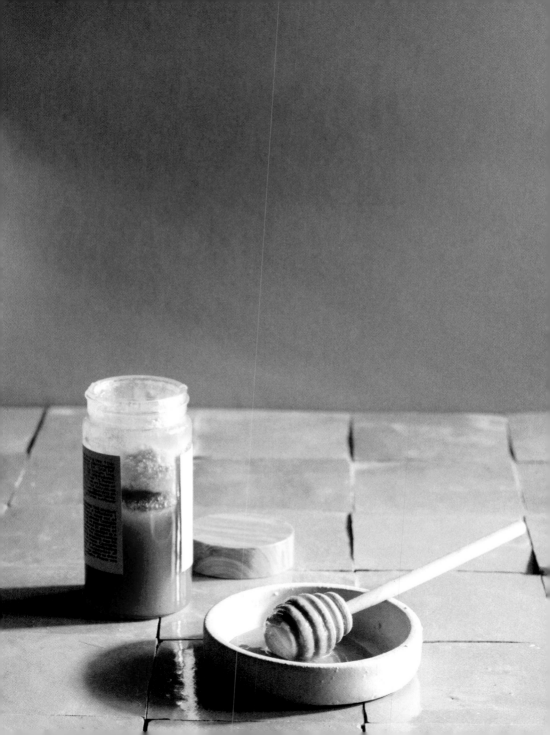

While boomers and seniors can benefit greatly from cannabis, obtaining suitable products may be challenging and uncomfortable. Walking into a dispensary for the first time may not be an older person's idea of a good time, even knowing it could result in an effective treatment for what ails them. If you are feeling trepidation about obtaining legal cannabis from a dispensary, you are not alone.

Do your homework and seek out a dispensary locally with a more sophisticated image or one that offers classes, particularly those geared toward older adults. Smart dispensary owners market to the AARP crowd or at senior centers to attract a more mature clientele. Bring a friend on your first trip to a dispensary. You may be surprised when you walk in to see a lot of customers with white and silver hair! Also, depending on where you live, such as some cities in California, you may be able to order cannabis products through a delivery service such as Eaze, Sava, and Goddess Delivers and have it brought right to your front door.

If you feel intimated by all the different product options, focus on the easiest to dose and consume: tablets or tinctures. Tablets will have little or no taste and will be precisely dosed, but tinctures may be preferable for taking a little more or a little less as needed. Review microdosing in chapter 8 as a good introduction to consuming THC for health and wellness purposes. If you're looking for relief from less acute conditions, ingesting a whole-plant CBD, oil-based tincture could be a gentler start but could also take days or weeks before you realize the effects.

For acute pain, vaping is a very rapid delivery method, but you may not like the idea of drawing anything into your lungs and your tolerance for smoke may have diminished with age. Tinctures, dissolvable tabs, sublingual or oral sprays, or even breath strips can be fast acting, particularly if infused with THC, and can be effective to reduce acute pain or anxiety quickly.

If you're an older individual interested in exploring cannabis or CBD for health and wellness, you may also be nervous about telling your family or friends. Chances are, with the changes in attitudes around cannabis, they will be more receptive than you think. Be open and honest with your loved ones and with your health care providers about your consumption so they can assist you as needed and make sure you don't take anything that might adversely affect any medications you are already taking.

If you are caring for someone older who could benefit from THC or CBD, introducing them to the idea of consuming could meet a lot of resistance. Provide them with reports or studies from sources they might recognize and trust, such as CNN or *Newsweek*. If they hear a high-profile figure promotes cannabis or CBD, it could also put them at ease. Let them know that Dr. Sanjay Gupta, Bill Gates, Morgan Freeman, Danny DeVito, Danny Glover, Patrick Stewart, Montel Williams, Melissa Etheridge, Whoopi Goldberg, Susan Sarandon, Frances McDormand, Rick Steves, and Ben & Jerry, the innovative ice-cream entrepreneurs, are all supporters of cannabis legalization and consumption for medical use, recreational use, or both.

Once again, we repeat that cannabis is not a cure-all. As you grow older and are prescribed multiple medications, you may find that the therapeutic use of cannabis and CBD can alleviate symptoms of aging and other ailments. Make sure that neither cannabis nor CBD interacts negatively with other medications you are taking. By introducing cannabis and CBD into your health care practices, you could reduce the need for multiple medications and lead a happier and healthier life.

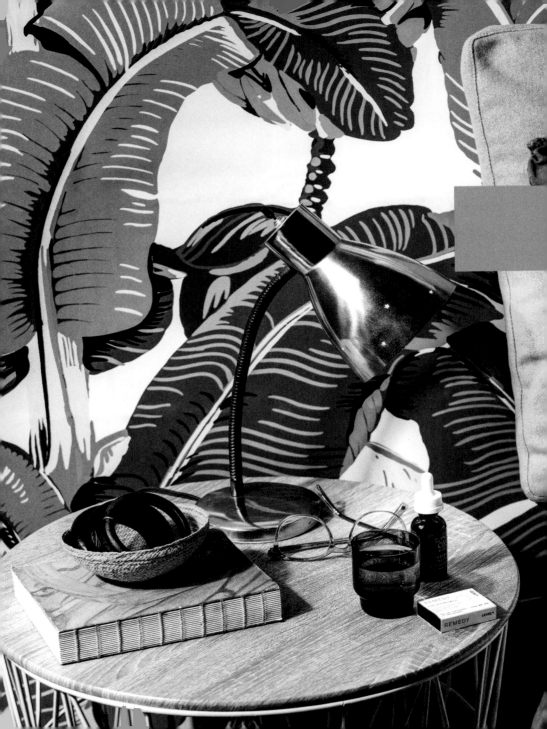

CHAPTER 13

Cannabis at Home

We've said it before: we believe someday cannabis will be in everyone's medicine chests like it used to be. As more governments legalize cannabis and CBD, all of us are faced with the prospect of bringing cannabis into our homes for recreation, health, and wellness, or all of the above.

In this book, we don't address cannabis use for treating children with epilepsy or other neurological brain conditions, although this is something some families are exploring. The legal and medical issues surrounding treating kids with cannabis are too complex and would take up an entire book, although you can find many resources online covering these topics.

In this final chapter, we'll address how to use cannabis at home safely and responsibly to gain the health and wellness benefits from the plant without endangering anyone in your household.

HAVING THE CONVERSATION

We both advocate engaging in an open dialogue about cannabis with members of your household, with an emphasis on scientific research and accurate, straightforward information. Having conversations about cannabis with everyone in your home is critical to creating a safe environment. Education can also help reduce anxiety associated with any residual stigma around cannabis or fear of the unfamiliar.

Start the process of bringing cannabis into your home by speaking with the adults. Whether you are living with a roommate, partner, spouse, parent, relative, or friend, come up with a plan together for keeping cannabis out of reach of children or anyone not wanting to accidentally consume a cannabis-infused product. Make a plan for properly storing and labeling cannabis products so the medicated chocolate bar sitting in the fridge doesn't end up in the wrong hands—and stomach.

If there are children in your home, the next step is deciding how to address the topic of cannabis with them. Too often, we wait to talk to our kids about drugs around the same time we talk to them about sex, picking the right time based on when we think they might encounter the topic at school or among their peers. Nowadays, talking about cannabis should be done with children of any age as part of normal conversation but always in an age-appropriate manner.

Refer to the medicinal plant as cannabis rather than marijuana or some other slang term. You can also call it *medicine* to use a term familiar to children. Treating cannabis in the home more like you treat over-the-counter or prescription medications is a more accurate alignment than calling it a drug. The goal is to make cannabis more normal and less scary.

Explain to your kids that adults are allowed to—or will be allowed to—use cannabis depending on the laws where you live. If your kids are older—preteens or teens—acknowledge that even though the legal age in your city, state, province, or country is eighteen, nineteen, or twenty-one, they should wait until their brains are fully formed. Neuroscientists say human brains are fully formed around twenty-five years of age.

With older kids, you can take a more candid approach and encourage them to come to you first for additional facts if they think they want to try cannabis sooner. The key is to not make cannabis forbidden, mysterious, or something they will want try in order to rebel. The conversations around cannabis in your home should be as normal as telling kids to stay out of the medicine chest and to not take medicine that isn't meant for them.

As we mentioned, the language you use for a candid conversation about cannabis with your kids should be age-appropriate. Any school-aged child will be hearing things from their peers or seeing things online about cannabis so start out by saying, "I want to talk with you about cannabis. What do you know about it?" Let them guide the conversation with their answers. Gauge their knowledge level, then go into a basic explanation about cannabis based on what they say they know and what you think they should know.

Find age-appropriate educational videos online that lay out the basics of how cannabis is medicine and why it is helpful to people for health and wellness. Don't compare cannabis to other drugs or perpetuate the myth that using cannabis leads to harder drugs. Let your kids ask any questions they have, and respond patiently and without judgment. Kids need to see that it is no big deal to talk about cannabis with you and that you are willing and able to speak with them about it in a relaxed and nonjudgmental manner.

Another conversation you might have is with the parents of kids coming over to your house or with houseguests. If you are confident that your cannabis products are securely stored, you may not need to broach the topic. Most people don't reveal an inventory of alcoholic products they have in their home or how they store it when someone is coming over or staying in the home. Because cannabis is safer than alcohol, there isn't any compelling reason why you would need to talk about your private consumption as long as you follow stringent safety measures. If the topic comes up or if you are asked directly, you can assure another parent that alcohol, medication, cannabis, and any other substances are kept out of reach or stored under lock and key.

USING CANNABIS AROUND YOUR KIDS

Whether or not you should consume cannabis in front of your kids depends on a number of factors, including their age and ability to understand what you are doing. If you are using cannabis for health reasons, taking the proper dosage and at the appropriate times of day or night is important to show your kids that cannabis is medicine. If you're using it as a sleep aid, for example, nighttime use after the kids are asleep makes sense. If you use it for destressing or recreation, consuming cannabis should look as normal as having a glass of wine or beer and, similarly, should not be consumed in excess.

If you smoke cannabis, don't do it around your kids because of the dangers of secondhand smoke. Consider other forms of consumption that can provide you with the desired effects without harmful by-products. Consume cannabis responsibly and know how your body and brain react to it so you are able to respond to your children's needs at all times.

Some parents we know keep various cannabis accessories out in the open around their houses. While each family has their own set of rules and comfort levels, be careful if you are using glass, ceramic, or otherwise breakable accessories. Keep them out of reach of small children who might knock them over and hurt themselves. Watch out for anything combustible you might be using for your cannabis consumption. Matches, lighters, or butane torches can land in the wrong hands with disastrous results.

Other than kids, using cannabis with houseguests or other adults in the home who don't consume is something that you should consider before doing. Only you know how you feel and react while using cannabis. If a situation requires careful attention or involves the use of machinery or anything needing balance and dexterity or fast reflexes, think twice before consuming unless you are microdosing and are not consuming to be in a heavily altered state of mind. Do not drive while under the influence of THC.

STORING CANNABIS SECURELY AT HOME

To keep cannabis out of reach of children or the unsuspecting guest, use some of the same techniques you use to keep your kids from accessing prescription or over-the-counter medicines with a few more security measures in place. Treat cannabis as you would any prescription drug, alcohol, cleaning product, or other substance that can be toxic to children and pets. Keep it out of reach, then go the extra step of locking it up.

Invest in a lockable storage bag or box for extra security and peace of mind when keeping cannabis in the home. There are many discreet and even designer lockable stash boxes and bags on the market that you can use to keep your cannabis tools out of reach of children. Cannabis flower is kept freshest in airtight containers that shut out light, such as a silicone jar, colored glass bottle, or metal box. You can use any nonlockable but airtight container and store it in a larger lockable one. Concentrates and tinctures can degrade over time, so keeping them in the cartridge or bottle they come in, storing them in a lockable box, and placing in a cool, dry cupboard is helpful.

Typically you do not refrigerate tinctures, but you can freeze concentrates if you are very careful to keep out any humidity and prevent condensation. One simple technique for freezing concentrates is to wrap them in parchment paper, place them into a lockable freezer bag or vacuum seal it, and then put them into an airtight glass container. More often than not, you are not purchasing enough of a concentrated form of cannabis that it needs longer-term storage.

Edibles can keep for a few days to a week or two in the refrigerator or for several months in the freezer, but make sure to use a lockable container. Plastic is fine to use in the fridge or freezer, and as long as your edibles are individually sealed in airtight packaging, your lockable storage device does not have to be airtight.

Even if you have open conversations with your kids about cannabis, it should not be accessible to them regardless of their age. All edibles should be properly marked. Label your cannabis edibles and products, whether you make or purchase them, with the recognizable green cross symbol. The company Cannacals makes decals and transfers for cannabis containers and baked goods that are handy for labeling.

Regardless of how you might use cannabis, using safety measures and being present and clear headed when it counts is most important. Safety comes first.

Cannabis, CBD, and Your Pets

We've talked a lot about using cannabis or CBD for people, but what about our pets? The major cannabinoid receptors in our bodies are also found in mammals, birds, reptiles, and fish. While THC is not recommended for pets, CBD products exist specifically formulated for horses, dogs, and cats, in particular.

CBD products for pets are touted for hip- and joint-pain relief, anxiety relief, seizure reduction, easing pain from glaucoma, relaxation, even cancer support. CBD may be combined with turmeric, glucosamine, and chondroitin for hip and joint pain or ginger and oregano for relaxation. Products often come as oils or capsules taken orally, topical creams to apply to aching muscles and joints, and edible treats such as chews and biscuits.

Do not give your pet a human dose of CBD. Speak with your vet first, and if they are not knowledgeable or receptive to CBD use, seek out a holistic vet who is.

THC can be toxic to your pet depending on their size and how much THC they consume. If your pet accidentally consumes cannabis products with high THC content, contact your veterinarian immediately. You can induce vomiting or give your pet activated charcoal tablets to try to reduce the effects of the THC. Aim for a healthy pet, not a high one!

AT THE END OF THE DAY

Our goal for writing this book wasn't to tell you that cannabis is the cure for your all ills—that is by no means true. The reason this book exists is because there is too much misinformation out there about cannabis. Opting to use cannabis is a personal choice, as is why and how you use it. While cannabis can be consumed socially, taking it for health and wellness is often a much more private and intimate process. Where you live usually dictates whether or not you can legally access and use cannabis.

We hope this book opens your eyes to the science behind the cannabis plant and how—and why—it affects your body and brain. Being a healthy, happy, and relaxed human being is a good thing no matter how you look at it. As we've detailed, cannabis could effectively address physical and mental conditions that impede your quality of life as well as nourish and fortify you to better deal with life's stressors. At the end of the day, what more could you ask for?

Acknowledgments

We could not have written this book without our personal cheerleaders and our professional colleagues who rallied behind us and who work daily to help people everywhere heal through the mindful use of cannabis.

A high five and warm embrace to our steadfast, talented book assistant, Kait Heacock.

A heartfelt thanks to the team at Ten Speed Press, including Julie Bennett, Ashley Pierce, Ashley Lima, Emma Campion, Windy Dorresteyn, David Hawk, Dan Myers, and Aaron Wehner.

FROM ALIZA

Thanks to my loving, patient family: Greg, Noa, and Josiah, as well as my uber supportive Ellementa business partners and dear friends, Melissa Pierce and Ashley Kingsley, and Ellementa team and local leaders. Could not have done this without you. Also special thanks to Dr. Robert Flannery (Dr. Robb) for his expertise and to the folks at Hey Lo for their terpene tips.

FROM JUNELLA

To my family and children, for their patience, wisdom, and loving encouragement. Thank you for supporting me in everything I do. I would like to extend a sincere gratitude to my patients, and am grateful for the extraordinary generosity that I received from those who let me share their stories about experiences with medications.

About the Authors

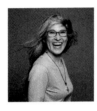

ALIZA SHERMAN is the cofounder of Ellementa, the fastest-growing women's network focused on health, wellness, and cannabis. She is the author of twelve books and has been featured in *USA Today*, *U.S. News & World Report*, *People*, *Time*, *Newsweek*, *Fast Company*, and *Forbes* and on CNN and CNBC.

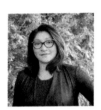

DR. JUNELLA CHIN is an osteopathic physician, the founder and chief medical officer of MedLeafRX (an integrative medicine practice based in California and New York), and director of education for the Association of Cannabis Specialists. She has been featured by St. Jude Medical, Cornell Tech, *USA Today*, and NBC's *Today* and has been an advocate for better understanding of the science and medicine of marijuana for over a decade.

Selected Bibliography

Aamodt, Sandra, interview by Tony Cox, "Brain Maturity Extends Well Beyond Teen Years." National Public Radio, October 10, 2011, www.npr.org/templates/story/story.php?storyId=141164708.

Aldrich, Michael R. "Tantric Cannabis Use in India." *Journal of Psychedelic Drugs* 9, no. 3 (1977): 227–233, doi:10.1080/02791072.1977.10472053.

Armstrong, Blake. "How Much CBD Should I Give My Dog?" *Cannabis for Pets*, cannabissupplementsforpets.com/cbd-oil-dosage-for-dogs-and-cats.

Ashton, Heather. "Adverse Effects of Cannabis." *Adverse Drug Reaction Bulletin*, 216, (2002): 827–830.

Ben-Shabat, Shimon, et al. "An Entourage Effect: Inactive Endogenous Fatty Acid Glycerol Esters Enhance 2-Arachidonoyl-Glycerol Cannabinoid Activity." *European Journal of Pharmacology* 353, no. 1 (1998): 23–31, doi:10.1016/s0014-2999(98)00392-6.

Bluett, R.J., et al. "Central Anandamide Deficiency Predicts Stress-Induced Anxiety: Behavioral Reversal through Endocannabinoid Augmentation." *Translational Psychiatry* 4, no. 7 (2014) doi:10.1038/tp.2014.53.

Cabral, G. A. and L. Griffin-Thomas. "Emerging Role of the CB2 Cannabinoid Receptor in Immune Regulation and Therapeutic Prospects." *Expert Reviews in Molecular Medicine*, U.S. National Library of Medicine, January 20, 2009, www.ncbi.nlm.nih.gov/pmc/articles/PMC2768535.

"Cannabinoid Nanoparticles, Hydrogel Combo Bolster Glaucoma Drops?" *American Optometric Association*, April 20, 2018, www.aoa.org/news/clinical-eye-care/glaucoma-cannabinoid-np-drop.

"Cannabis as Medicine? More and More Baby Boomers Think So." *The Spokesman-Review*, August 17, 2018, www.spokesman.com/stories/2018/aug/12/baby-boomers-turning-cannabis-medicine.

"Cannabis Use and Youth: A Parent's Guide." *What's the Difference between Anxiety and Stress?*, www.heretohelp.bc.ca/workbook/cannabis-use-and-youth-a-parents-guide.

"Cannabis Use, Cautions, Contraindications." *Medicinal Cannabis*, October 3, 2010, medicalcbd.wordpress.com/marijuana-use-cautions-and-contraindications.

Childs, Emma, et al. "Dose-Related Effects of Delta-9-THC on Emotional Responses to Acute Psychosocial Stress." *Drug and Alcohol Dependence* 177 (2017): 136–144, doi:10.1016/j.drugalcdep.2017.03.030.

Dittner, Antonia. "Cognitive-Behavioural Therapy (CBT) for Adult Attention Deficit Hyperactivity Disorder (ADHD): a Randomised Controlled Trial." doi.org/10.1186/ISRCTN03732556.

Dlugos, Andrea, et al. "Acute Stress Increases Circulating Anandamide and Other N-Acylethanolamines in Healthy Humans." *Neuropsychopharmacology* 37, no. 11 (2012): 2416–2427, doi:10.1038/npp.2012.100.

Fernández-Ruiz, Javier, et al. "Cannabidiol for Neurodegenerative Disorders: Important New Clinical Applications for This Phytocannabinoid?" *British Journal of Clinical Pharmacology* 75, no. 2 (2013) 323–333, doi:10.1111/j.1365-2125.2012.04341.x.

Fine, Perry G., and Mark J. Rosenfeld. "The Endocannabinoid System, Cannabinoids, and Pain." *Rambam Maimonides Medical Journal*, 4, no. 4 (2013) doi:10.5041/rmmj.10129.

Gable, Robert S. "Comparison of Acute Lethal Toxicity of Commonly Abused Psychoactive Substances." *Addiction*, 99, no. 6 (2004) 686–696, doi:10.1111/j.1360-0443.2004.00744.x.

Gertsch, J., et al. "Phytocannabinoids beyond the Cannabis Plant—Do They Exist?" *British Journal of Pharmacology*, U.S. National Library of Medicine, (2010): 523–529 www.ncbi.nlm.nih.gov/pubmed/20590562.

Gordon, Serena. "Medical Marijuana a Hit with Seniors." *Consumer HealthDay*, July 5, 2018, consumer.healthday.com/public-health-information-30/marijuana-news-759/medical-marijuana-a-hit-with-seniors-735432.html.

"GPCR." *Nature News*, Nature Publishing Group, 2014, www.nature.com/scitable/ebooks/essentials-of-cell-biology-14749010/122997540.

Head, Kathi. "Endocannabinoid System 101." *Take 5 Daily*, Thorne Magazine, April 6, 2018, www.thorne.com/take-5-daily/article/endocannabinoid-system-101.

Hill, Kevin P., et al. "Cannabis and Pain: A Clinical Review." *Cannabis and Cannabinoid Research* 2, no. 1 (2017): 96–104, doi:10.1089/can.2017.0017.

Hossain, Mohammad, et al. "Chemical Analysis of Extracts from Newfoundland Berries and Potential Neuroprotective Effects." *Antioxidants*, 5, no. 4 (2016): 36, doi:10.3390/antiox5040036.

Howlett, Allyn, et al. "CB1 Cannabinoid Receptors and Their Associated Proteins." *Current Medicinal Chemistry*, 17, no. 14 (2010): 1382–1393, doi:10.2174/092986710790980023.

"How Your Endocannabinoid System Can Jump Start Your Sex Life." *Emerald Health Bioceuticals*, emeraldhealthbio.com/blogs/news/how-your-endocannabinoid-system-can-jump-start-your-sex-life.

Isakson, Peter. "Cyclooxygenase-2: A Novel Target for Safer Anti-Inflammatory Drugs." *Side Effects of Anti-Inflammatory Drugs IV* (1997): 339–340, doi:10.1007/978-94-011-5394-2_48.

Jacques, Jacqueline. "Understanding the Phytocannabinoids." *Take 5 Daily: A Thorne Magazine*, May 11, 2018, www.thorne.com/take-5-daily/article/understanding-the-phytocannabinoids.

Johnson, Renée. *Hemp as an Agricultural Commodity*. Congressional Research Service, 2018.

Johnson, Sara B., et al. "Adolescent Maturity and the Brain: The Promise and Pitfalls of Neuroscience Research in Adolescent Health Policy." *Journal of Adolescent Health* 45, no. 3 (2009): 216–221, doi:10.1016/j.jadohealth.2009.05.016.

Katchan, Valeria, et al. "Cannabinoids and Autoimmune Diseases: A Systematic Review." *Autoimmunity Reviews*, 15, no. 6 (2016): 513–528, doi:10.1016/j.autrev.2016.02.008.

Komorowski, J., and H Stepień. "The Role of the Endocannabinoid System in the Regulation of Endocrine Function and in the Control of Energy Balance in Humans." *Postepy Higieny i Medycyny Doswiadczalnej (Online)*, U.S. National Library of Medicine, (2007) www.ncbi.nlm.nih.gov/pubmed/17369778.

Krier, Joel, et al. "Reclassification of Genetic-Based Risk Predictions as GWAS Data Accumulate." *Genome Medicine* 8, no. 1 (2016) doi:10.1186/s13073-016-0272-5.

Larsen, Dana. "Canada's Shocking Waste of Medical Cannabis." *Vancouver Sun*, July 7, 2014, vancouversun.com/news/community-blogs/canadas-shocking-waste-of-medical-cannabis.

"Learn About Terpenes." *SC Labs*, www.sclabs.com/terpenes.

Lee, Martin A. "Single Compound vs. Whole Plant CBD." *Project CBD: Medical Marijuana & Cannabinoid Science*, February 22, 2015, www.projectcbd.org/science/cannabis-pharmacology/single-compound-vs-whole-plant-cbd.

Lloyd, Shawnta L., and Catherine W. Striley. "Marijuana Use Among Adults 50 Years or Older in the 21st Century." *Gerontology and Geriatric Medicine* 4, (2018): 233372141878166, doi:10.1177/2333721418781668.

Mackie, Kenneth. "Faculty of 1000 Evaluation for Reversible and Regionally Selective Downregulation of Brain Cannabinoid CB(1) Receptors in Chronic Daily Cannabis Smokers." *F1000—Post-Publication Peer Review of the Biomedical Literature*, 2011, doi:10.3410 /f.12160957.13320055.

"Marijuana Use Continues to Grow among Baby Boomers." *ScienceDaily*, September 6, 2018, www.sciencedaily.com/releases/ 2018/09/180906100458.htm.

"Medical Marijuana Could Reduce Opioid Use in Older Adults, Study Finds." *Culture of C.A.R.E. | Northwell Health*, www.northwell.edu/about/ news/press-releases/medical-marijuana-could-reduce-opioid-use-older-adults-study-finds.

"Medicinal Properties of Terpenes Found in Cannabis Sativa and Humulus Lupulus." *NeuroImage*, Academic Press, August 4, 2018, www.sciencedirect.com/science/article/pii/ S0223523418306408.

Naidu, P. S., et al. "Synergy between Enzyme Inhibitors of Fatty Acid Amide Hydrolase and Cyclooxygenase in Visceral Nociception." *Journal of Pharmacology and Experimental Therapeutics* 329, no. 1 (2008): 48–56, doi: 10.1124/jpet.108.143487.

Nelson, Kristine A, and Declan Walsh. "The Use of Cannabinoids in Palliative Medicine." *Progress in Palliative Care* 6, no. 5 (1998): 160–163, doi: 10.1080/09699260.1998.11746811.

Niazy, Esmail M. "Influence of Oleic Acid and Other Permeation Promoters on Transdermal Delivery of Dihydroergotamine through Rabbit Skin." *International Journal of Pharmaceutics*, 67, no. 1 (1991): 97–100, doi:10.1016/0378-5173(91)90269-t.

NYU Langone Medical Center. "Brain-imaging study links cannabinoid receptors to post-traumatic stress disorder: First pharmaceutical treatment for PTSD within reach." *ScienceDaily*, May 14, 2013, *www.sciencedaily.com/ releases/2013/05/130514085016.htm*.

Oláh, Attila, et al. "Targeting Cannabinoid Signaling in the Immune System: 'High'-Ly Exciting Questions, Possibilities, and Challenges." *Frontiers in Immunology*, 8 (2017): doi:10.3389/fimmu.2017.01487.

"Opioid Overdose." Centers for Disease Control and Prevention, August 30, 2017, www.cdc.gov/ drugoverdose/data/prescribing.html.

Pacher, Pal, et al. "The Endocannabinoid System as an Emerging Target of Pharmacotherapy." *Pharmacological Reviews*, U.S. National Library of Medicine, September 2006, www.ncbi.nlm .nih.gov/pmc/articles/PMC2241751/.

Parker, Linda A, et al. "Regulation of Nausea and Vomiting by Cannabinoids." *British Journal of Pharmacology* 163, no. 7 (2011): 1411–1422, doi:10.1111/j.1476-5381.2010.01176.x.

Pertwee, Roger G. "Cannabinoid Pharmacology: The First 66 Years." *British Journal of Pharmacology*, Nature Publishing Group, January 2006, www.ncbi.nlm.nih.gov/pmc/ articles/PMC1760722/.

"Plants Other Than Cannabis That Produce Cannabinoids." *Royal Queen Seeds*, December 8, 2017, www.royalqueenseeds.com/blog-plants-other-than-cannabis-that-produce-cannabinoids-n714.

Prasanthi, D., and Pk Lakshmi. "Terpenes: Effect of Lipophilicity in Enhancing Transdermal Delivery of Alfuzosin Hydrochloride." *Journal of Advanced Pharmaceutical Technology & Research* 3, no. 4 (2012): 216, doi:10.4103/2231-4040.104712.

Rieder, Michael J. "Is the Medical Use of Cannabis a Therapeutic Option for Children?" *Paediatrics & Child Health* 21, no. 1 (2016): 31–34, doi:10.1093/pch/21.1.31.

Russo, Ethan B., et al. "Phytochemical and Genetic Analyses of Ancient Cannabis from Central Asia." *Journal of Experimental Botany* 59, no. 15 (2008): 4171–4182, doi:10.1093/jxb/ ern260.

Russo, Ethan. "Cannabinoids in the Management of Difficult to Treat Pain." *Therapeutics and Clinical Risk Management* 4 (2008): 245–259, doi:10.2147/tcrm.s1928.

Russo, Ethan. "Cannabis Treatments in Obstetrics and Gynecology: A Historical Review." *Journal of Cannabis Therapeutics*, 2, no. 3–4 (2002): 5–35, doi:10.1300/ j175v02n03_02.

Russo, Ethan B. "Taming THC: Potential Cannabis Synergy and Phytocannabinoid-Terpenoid Entourage Effects." *British Journal of Pharmacology*, 163, no. 7 (2011) 1344–1364, doi:10.1111/j.1476-5381.2011.01238.x.

Schug, Stephan. "Faculty of 1000 Evaluation for Efficacy and Adverse Effects of Buprenorphine in Acute Pain Management: Systematic Review and Meta-Analysis of Randomised Controlled Trials." *F1000—Post-Publication Peer Review of the Biomedical Literature*, 2018, doi:10.3410/f.732927620.793546380.

Sharma, Charu, et al. "Small Molecules from Nature Targeting G-Protein Coupled Cannabinoid Receptors: Potential Leads for Drug Discovery and Development." *Evidence-Based Complementary and Alternative Medicine*, 2015 (2015): 1–26, doi:10.1155/2015/238482.

Sulak, Dustin. "NORML—Working to Reform Marijuana Laws." *The National Organization for the Reform of Marijuana Laws*, norml.org/library/item/introduction-to-the-endocannabinoid-system.

Sun, Andrew J., and Michael L. Eisenberg. "Association Between Marijuana Use and Sexual Frequency in the United States: A Population-Based Study." *The Journal of Sexual Medicine* 14, no. 11 (2017): 1342–1347, doi:10.1016/j.jsxm.2017.09.005.

Tambaro, Simone, and Marco Bortolato. "Cannabinoid-Related Agents in the Treatment of Anxiety Disorders: Current Knowledge and Future Perspectives." *Recent Patents on CNS Drug Discovery* 7, no. 1 (2012): 25–40, doi:10.2174/157488912798842269.

Turner, S. E., et al. "Molecular Pharmacology of Phytocannabinoids." *Progress in the Chemistry of Organic Natural Products*, U.S. National Library of Medicine, 2017, www.ncbi.nlm.nih.gov/pubmed/28120231.

Tzadok, Michal, et al. "CBD-Enriched Medical Cannabis for Intractable Pediatric Epilepsy." *Seizure* 35 (2016): 41–44, doi:10.1016/j.seizure.2016.01.004.

Vinod, K. Yaragudri, and Basalingappa L. Hungund. "Role of the Endocannabinoid System in Depression and Suicide." *Trends in Pharmacological Sciences* 27, no. 10 (2006): 539–545, doi:10.1016/j.tips.2006.08.006.

Wang, D. "The Essential Role of G Protein-Coupled Receptor (GPCR) Signaling in Regulating T Cell Immunity." *Immunopharmacology and Immunotoxicology*, U.S. National Library of Medicine (June 2018), www.ncbi.nlm.nih.gov/pubmed/29433403.

Ward, Sara Jane, and Ellen A. Walker. "Sex and Cannabinoid CB1 Genotype Differentiate Palatable Food and Cocaine Self-Administration Behaviors in Mice." *Behavioural Pharmacology* 20, no. 7 (2009): 605–613, doi:10.1097/fbp.0b013e328331ba30.

Wu, Brian. "Marijuana and Erectile Dysfunction: What Is the Connection?" *Medical News Today*, MediLexicon International, August 9, 2018, www.medicalnewstoday.com/articles/317104.php.

Index

A

ADHD (attention deficit/hyperactivity disorder), 132, 134–35
aging, 146, 148–49
alpha-pinene, 52
anandamide, 35, 126, 128
ankylosing spondylitis (AS), 3–4
Anslinger, Harry Jacob, 14
anxiety, 108–10
APIs (active pharmaceutical ingredients), 89
appetite
    increasing, 122–23, 142
    suppressing, 142
autoimmune disorders, 120–22

B

beta-pinene, 52
beverages, 71, 81–82, 96
bongs, 77
bud, 65–66
butane hash oil (BHO), 67

C

cancer, 122–23
cannabinoids
    boiling points of, 79
    CB1 and CB2 receptors and, 32
    entourage effect and, 42–43
    finding specific, 38
    isolating, 42–43

number of, 32, 35
overviews of specific, 38–41, 44
relationships among, 36–37
research on, 36
terpenes and, 51
See also individual cannabinoids
cannabis
    acute conditions and, 105–12
    children and, 134, 151–56
    chronic conditions and, 115–23
    delivery methods for, 73–82, 84–87, 89–91
    dosing, 93–100, 102
    forms of, 61, 65–68, 71
    history of, 9–15
    legalization of, 1–2
    medications and, 2
    mental conditions and, 125–32, 134–35
    misconceptions about, 1, 4, 9, 158
    "overdose" of, 13
    pets and, 157
    for recreational use, 145–46
    research on, 1
    seniors and, 146, 148–49
    storing, 155–56
    talking about, 152–54
    terpenes and, 49–52, 54–58
    well-being and, 137–46, 148–49
    whole-plant extracts vs. isolates, 42–43

Cannabis indica, 18, 21
cannabis plants
    cultivars of, 19
    growing, 22, 62
    harvesting and processing, 62–64
    pesticides and, 22, 62
    scientific classification of, 17–18, 21–22
    strains of, 18–19
    trichomes on, 23
Cannabis ruderalis, 18, 22
Cannabis sativa, 18, 21, 46
capsules, 82, 97
carbs, 76
caryophyllene, 54, 79
cats, 157
CBC (cannabichromene), 44
CBD (cannabidiol)
    boiling point of, 79
    cannabis- vs. hemp-derived, 46–47
    CB1 and CB2 receptors and, 32
    microdosing, 93–100, 102
    pets and, 157
    potential therapeutic benefits of, 44
    psychoactive nature of, 19, 41
    in raw cannabis leaves, 74
    THC and, 41, 42
CBG (cannabigerol), 36, 37, 44
CBGA (cannabigerol acid), 36, 37, 38
CBN (cannabinol), 37, 40, 79